# Holding the Tiger's Tail

An Acupuncture Techniques Manual
in the
Treatment of Disease

—

Skya Gardner-Abbate

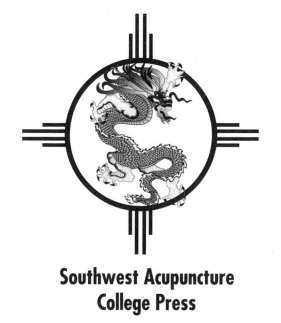

**Southwest Acupuncture
College Press**

Holding the Tiger's Tail
An Acupuncture Techniques Manual in the
Treatment of Disease
by Skya Gardner-Abbate

ISBN# 0-9628620-1-0
Library of Congress #96-067830

Publisher: Southwest Acupuncture College Press
325 Paseo de Peralta, Suite 500
Santa Fe, New Mexico, 87501, U.S.A.

To my teachers at Hepingli and Beida Hospitals, Beijing, China, for their patience and generosity in sharing their clinical knowledge with me in the summers of 1988 and 1989.

To the graduates of the classes of 1988 through 1996 at Southwest Acupuncture College for graciously giving me the opportunity to refine my clinical skills and develop this book by teaching them the techniques I acquired in China and then polished in private practice.

To my husband, Anthony, my inspiration.

# Credits

Cover concept and design by Anthony Abbate

Cover and Part illustrations by Tōru Miyake

Edited by Lawrence Grinnell

Illustrations by Christine R. Oagley

Photos by Jill Fineberg

Foreword by Giovanni Maciocia, C.Ac. (Nanjing)

# Acknowledgments

The production of a book involves more than the thoughts of an author. Many people are involved in the process of bringing those thoughts to the readers. The following people were not only instrumental but also invaluable in assisting me in the vision that is this book.

With grateful acknowledgment to my editor, Lawrence Grinnell, who patiently processed and clarified my thoughts so this book would be not only possible but also pleasurable to read.

To Tōru Miyake for his masterful grasp of the spirit of the tiger, as shown in his traditional paper cuts on the cover and within the book.

To Christine Oagley for her creativity and conscientiousness in materializing the energetic concepts of Chinese medicine in her illustrations.

To Cindy Wolf for her endless tenacity and computer expertise in formatting the tables and figures for me.

To Christine Arundell for her impeccable ability in editorial assistance.

To Bobbi Anaya for doing not only her job as an administrator but additionally acting as the liaison between me and all the other people involved in this book.

To Jill Fineberg for her playful spirit in photographing some pretty strange things!

To all of you, thank you so very much for your endless help in making this book a reality.

# Appendix

## Translations of the Point Names

## Figures and Photographs

## Tables

# FOREWORD

**A** good diagnosis is only the first step in a successful acupuncture treatment. After diagnosing, we should select a correct treatment principle, choose appropriate points in the right combination, apply the correct needling technique, retain the needles for an optimum time, and finally, withdraw the needles properly. Although several books illustrate the art of diagnosis, few have concentrated on the arts of point selection and needling technique. Skya Gardner-Abbate's book fills these gaps admirably. Her teaching and clinical experience breathe from every page and bring the book to life. Her teaching experience has obviously given her an insight into the needs and questions of acupuncture students, which the book answers in a clear and lively manner. As well, her clinical experience solidly illustrates and underpins the theories expounded.

Acupuncture has a rich variety of styles, e.g., Japanese acupuncture, so-called TCM acupuncture, Five Element acupuncture, Korean acupuncture, ear acupuncture, micro-systems acupuncture, myo-facial acupuncture, and many others. This book goes beyond such categorization and encompasses all styles by going to the heart of acupuncture and into the nature of points, thus transcending the differences among various acupuncture methods. For these reasons, her book will appeal to all practitioners of acupuncture, no matter what style they practice. For example, the tables in the book contain invaluable clinical information. They including twenty-two methods of tonification and sedation of points, the signs of point pathology (never seen before in an acupuncture book), clinical use of the Five Shu points and points of the Extraordinary Vessels, the clinical use of the Luo points, rules of point selection, needling strategies, clinical use of the Xi (cleft) points, techniques and depths of insertion of needles, bloodletting techniques for blood stasis patterns in the occipital area, clinical use of the Plum Blossom needle, and many others. I predict that such tables will be an inestimable aid to both students and practitioners.

In the process of adapting a foreign system of medicine, such as that of Chinese medicine in the West, the acquiring culture goes through various stages. The first is to translate the other culture's medical texts. After some time, the new culture adapts the foreign medical culture, thus making it its own; this is a stage of maturity in the assimilation of another medical culture. Skya Gardner-Abbate's book reflects an increasing adaptation of acupuncture to Western clinical conditions, contributing to a process that will eventually lead to the birth of a cosmopolitan and truly international medicine.

GIOVANNI MACIOCIA

# PREFACE

As I write this book, acupuncture and its associated modalities have been thoroughly institutionalized in formal schools of acupuncture in the United States for approximately twenty years. The schools pursue their mission and generally succeed in giving a basic acupuncture education. On the whole, they produce well-rounded, competent healthcare providers who are not only skilled in acupuncture but also in other branches of the Oriental medical arts as well, that is, nutrition, exercise/breathing therapy (Tai ji/Qi gong), massage/bone-soft tissue manipulation (Tuina), and Chinese herbal medicine.

Gradually, the scope of the practice of American acupuncture is broadening to include the full range of Oriental therapeutic modalities. So also, improved clinical practice demands that the depth of training in acupuncture techniques be explored for the benefit of the patient and the recognition of Oriental medicine in the United States. Schools must teach the many techniques that have been developed over the centuries so that students can recognize and refine the appropriate treatment techniques for specific disease patterns.

In my opinion—based on an intimate fifteen-year association with the field of American acupuncture education, both as an instructor and an educational specialist—there appears to be a weakness in the curricula of the colleges in the area of acupuncture techniques. This deficiency can be explained from a number of perspectives, one of which is that this skill is a function of the amount of time that acupuncture has been in the United States. In addition, the constraints of time in student clinics—where so many tasks demand the attention of the novice—tend to limit the use of modalities other than needles and Chinese herbs. And, of course, the curriculum offered in schools is generally determined by which instructors are available and their expertise. Most teachers in American institutions are products of American schools. However, they also put in an unrelenting effort at self-education through books, journals, workshops, and foreign externships in Asia. They are therefore often at a point in their careers when they have greater expertise and have evolved into better teachers who have higher expectations for their students.

As the curricula at the master's level begins to stabilize throughout the country because of experience and nationally recognized guidelines, it is now the responsibility of the schools to cultivate their courses and to teach with greater precision and effectiveness. This is particularly true in the clinical context, the ultimate reality of the patient/practitioner interface. Teachers who have garnered valuable treatment techniques as a result of clinical experience and continued education must inspire students with their skills. The instructors must also demand a greater proficiency and closer correlation between acupuncture modalities and specific clinical conditions.

With these things in mind, I have written this book. The information presented here is primarily a synthesis of two experiences. First, I went on two China study tours specifically to accumulate knowledge about those techniques that enhance therapeutic effectiveness. The techniques were derived from and demonstrated in actual clinical practice. I have also used them in private practice and taught them to nine classes of graduates to assess their effectiveness. They have proven to be useful and efficient. Second, the balance of the book contains original work on specialized topics with which I have had extensive clinical experience.

Part I of this book outlines what could be termed general treatment strategies. These are thought processes and approaches to the practice of Chinese medicine and to general medical conditions, rather than to specific illnesses. Part II of the manual addresses the treatment of specific clinical conditions with assorted Oriental modalities. Actual case studies are included that illustrate the applications of the techniques presented.

This work is by no means intended to be a technique compendium. Rather, it is a beginning-to-midlevel manual that can provide students and practitioners with useful treatment strategies. I have written the book to stimulate teachers and clinicians to sharpen their diagnostic abilities and to coordinate diagnosis with clinically effective techniques. Simultaneously, I hope to challenge the reader to go beyond the simple and sometimes mindless insertion of a needle, to consciously hone and bring to full awareness the attention needed to skillfully and compassionately treat the complexity of the human condition.

To hold the needle as if holding the tiger's tail is a dangerous, magical, and powerful act. The willingness to accept this danger and opportunity is as necessary to treatment as it is to living. I urge all readers to "hold the tiger's tail."

SKYA GARDNER-ABBATE,
M.A., D.O.M., Dipl.Ac., Dipl.C.H.
Department of Clinical Medicine,
Southwest Acupuncture College
Sante Fe/Albuquerque, New Mexico
June, 1996

# GENERAL TREATMENT
# APPROACHES

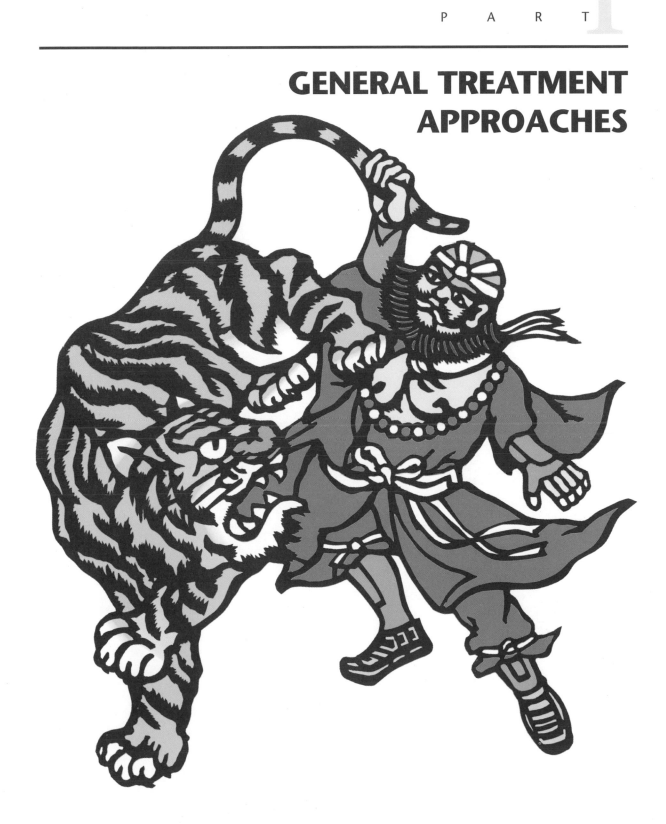

# THE RELATIONSHIP BETWEEN THE METHODS OF DIAGNOSIS AND THERAPEUTIC EFFECTIVENESS

Practitioners agree that the aim of every acupuncture treatment should be to restore balance and wholeness and thus to relieve the patient's "disease." In acupuncture, the ability to do this is ultimately through the needle. Thus, excellent needle technique is extremely important in the treatment process. Needless to say, even the best needle techniques cannot compensate for an inaccurate diagnosis or a faulty treatment plan, so these skills need to be equally developed. And the ability to arrive at a correct diagnosis is correspondingly dependent on the ability to collect the necessary diagnostic information through the classical methods of diagnosis: inspection, auscultation, olfaction, palpation, and inquiry. Also, the practitioner must be able to weave the signs and symptoms into a synergetic whole that portrays each individual's unique constellation of energy.

Within classical Chinese medicine there is an intrinsic diagnostic logic that pervades the process from the first gathering of data through to therapeutic effectiveness. These related steps are discussed here and summarized in *Table 1*, "Intake to Improvement: The Inherent Logic of the Chinese Diagnostic and Delivery Systems."

**Goal.**  Health of the patient.

**Step 1.**  Collect the data necessary to arrive at a diagnosis through inspection, auscultation, olfaction, palpation, and inquiry.  Together, these methods, organized around the senses, allow the practitioner to gather the fullest possible range of data.

**Step 2.**  Assess the situation, that is, organize the data into the appropriate and/or preferred diagnostic framework.  Each framework, like a lens, helps the practitioner to view the person from a unique perspective.  Preferred paradigms are often a function of how much exposure the practitioner has had to them.  Their effectiveness is directly linked to the ability of that paradigm to contribute to seeing the "picture" of the patient.

Pictures of reality, ways of viewing the world, can range from photographic preciseness to impressionistic imagery to the obscurity of modern art.  Each picture, like a paradigm, is a vision, no better and no worse than the other, simply a way of organizing experience.  Acupuncture paradigms, the "pictures" we use to organize our experience of the patient, include the following:

    a.  yin/yang
    b.  qi and blood
    c.  three treasures (qi, jing, shen)
    d.  four levels (wei, qi, ying, xue)
    e.  five elements (wood, fire, earth, metal, water)
    f.  six divisions (Taiyang, Shaoyang, Yangming, Taiyin, Shaoyin, Jueyin)
    g.  zang-fu
    h.  essential substances (qi, blood, body fluid, jing, shen, marrow)
    i.  eight principles (internal-external, excess-deficient, yin-yang, hot-cold)
    j.  extraordinary vessels
    k.  jing luo (meridian therapy)

l.  luo vessels

m.  San Jiao

n.  exogenous pathogens (wind, cold, damp, dryness, heat, summer-heat)

o.  endogenous pathogens (the emotions: anger, joy, fear, fright, grief, worry, and melancholy)

p.  miscellaneous pathogens (neither exogenous or endogenous, they include factors such as dietary indiscretions, exercise habits, trauma, scars, radiation, and so on)

q.  secondary pathological products (stagnant blood, damp-phlegm)

r.  energetic layers (skin, muscle, meridian, blood, organ, bone)

s.  Western medical model and its etiological factors

t.  Japanese systems

u.  palpatory findings

v.  heaven-man-earth

In order to come to a diagnosis, the practitioner must artistically and carefully weave the material data from the physical exam with the voluminous information revealed in the interview. Thus, a coherent and accurate assessment can be achieved. The interview process can give the practitioner and the patient a glimpse of the human spirit that underlies the context of any individual life. But it must be conducted with an openness and rapport that allows the richness as well as the sickness of the person to emerge. Likewise, if the meaning of the illness can be captured and conveyed to the patient, true healing can begin and both the patient and the practitioner can work together to remedy the disease. The questions should not become an obstacle to seeing who the person really is. The history, if clearly elicited, can be as therapeutic as the treatment itself.

**Step 3.** Identify the problem, that is, arrive at a diagnostic statement. Like an hypothesis, this statement is an educated guess, a tentative assumption based on facts, about what is going on with the person. It should be an artful, clear, simple statement, a summary of the patient's present as it relates to his or her past—for example, Liver blood deficiency that has become Liver qi stagnation.

The fact that a diagnosis is not final, just as no hypothesis is final until it has been verified, is an important guiding principle in treatment. The practitioner must evaluate this hypothesis and modify it every time the patient is seen.

**Step 4.** Formulate a treatment principle that is a therapeutic and educational plan directly related to the diagnosis. For example, a diagnostic statement of "Spleen qi deficiency" has a treatment plan of "tonify the qi of the Spleen."

**Step 5.** Select the appropriate treatment modalities that have known clinical effectiveness in treating the diagnosed condition. The most common modalities include, but are not limited to, the following:

  a.  acupuncture and its microsystems, such as auricular therapy, scalp acupuncture, hand acupuncture, and so on.
  b.  moxibustion
  c.  cupping
  d.  Plum Blossom needle therapy
  e.  gwa sha
  f.  herbal medicine
  g.  tuina
  h.  massage
  i.  nutritional therapy
  j.  exercise/breathing therapy
  k.  lifestyle changes

**Step 6.** If acupuncture is used, select the points to be needled. Provide the rationale for each point's use and determine the method of needling, that is, tonification or dispersion. For example, tonify BL 18 (Ganshu), Back Shu point of the Liver to nourish the Liver Blood and tonify LR 4 ( Zhongfeng), the metal point on the wood meridian to move the Liver qi stagnation, because metal controls wood.

**Step 7.** Administer treatment. Verify that there is a correlation between the treatment plan and what is actually done. That is, if the strategy is to tonify, make sure that the needle technique is indeed a tonification technique.

**Step 8.** Evaluate therapeutic effectiveness for the major complaint after administering each treatment.

**Step 9.** Continually reassess other active problems in subsequent visits.

*Table 1.* Intake to Improvement: The Inherent Logic of the Chinese Diagnostic and Delivery Systems

| GOAL | THE HEALTH OF PATIENT |
|---|---|
| Step 1 | Perform "the methods of diagnosis" |
| Step 2 | Organize the data into a diagnostic framework |
| Step 3 | Arrive at a diagnosis |
| Step 4 | Formulate a treatment principle |
| Step 5 | Select the appropriate treatment modality |
| Step 6 | Select the points to be needled Provide the rationale for each point's use, and determine the method of needling |
| Step 7 | Administer treatment |
| Step 8 | Evaluate therapeutic effectiveness |
| Step 9 | Continually reassess |

Although the steps detailed here are expressed linearly, they are actually cyclically related to each other. Each step leads to and prompts the next one, influencing it so the circle of wholeness and health is achieved. The interrelated steps bend into circles, all organized around the goal of treatment, which is to restore the patient to balance. Health is a reflection of that balance.  *(See Figure 1, Intake to Improvement:  The Cyclic Relationship of the Components of the Chinese Diagnostic and Delivery Systems.)*

This is the exquisite logic of Oriental medicine that must guide the practitioner in treatment.  If the results are not satisfactory, the practitioner is encouraged to look back at all of these steps to see if:

1.  They are all being performed to the best of one's ability.
2.  They are mutually related to each other.
3.  The intent is actually being achieved.  For instance, is a tonification or a dispersion technique being applied to the needle?

From the preface of this book and from its title, it should be clear that the focus is neither on how to perform the methods of diagnosis nor on what the data collected from these procedures mean.  Neither is it to explain how to plug that information into established diagnostic frameworks that dictate diagnoses and suggest treatment principles.  Rather, the theme of this book is how to select treatment modalities from the acupuncture techniques that have proven clinically effective in the treatment of select disease patterns with which I am familiar.

Still, it is imperative to remind practitioners that the diagnostic process is full of intricacies and that these can be controlled by healthcare providers.  This knowledge helps practitioners develop the ability to critique their performance so that the best interests of their patients are served.

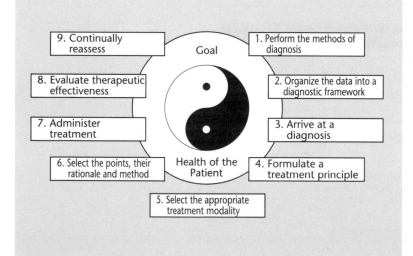

*Figure 1.*  Intake to Improvement:  The Cyclic Relationship of the Components of the Chinese Diagnostic and Delivery Systems

Practitioners also need to be mindful that the success of any treatment is not simply a function of the steps listed above, although these are critical variables. Experienced practitioners are aware that the practitioner/patient relationship is the context within which the delivery of healthcare is provided. This relationship, according to classical Chinese medicine, is not operating at its most effective level when it is only a mechanical process of gathering information and administering a treatment. A caring atmosphere of concern and confidentiality, mutual respect and rapport, professionalism and attention to the patient's presence is as meaningful to bringing the patient back to health and balance as the steps given in *Table 1*. The practitioner's belief in the medicine and in her or his own abilities are also empowering and will create a mindset where the patient receives the best the practitioner has to give.

If we agree with the *Neijing* that healing represents a change and moves the patient's spirit,[1] then there are almost unlimited modalities to effect that change. Obviously, acupuncture is a powerful healing tool and the allied Chinese medical arts are also effective as both independent and supplementary modalities. But sometimes such change can be elicited from touch, talk, and laughter, in short, from the ability of the practitioner to engage the patient's spirit. The highest level of the practice of healing, then, is not exclusively the logical aspect of diagnosis and treatment but the ability of one human spirit to make meaningful contact with another. As such, healing is a sacred and noble endeavor.

*Case 1* provides an example of the complexity of the diagnostic and delivery system.

---

1. Larée C and Rochat de la Vallee E: The practitioner-patient relationship: wisdom from the Chinese classics. *J Trad Acu,* Winter, 1990-91; 14–17, 48–50.

## Case 1. Pulses at the adaptive level

The reading of emotions through the pulse had never been my focus until the following case. True, I had always noticed a strong correlation between grief and Lung pulses as well as between fear and Kidney pulses. Of course, a particularly wiry pulse seemed to have aggravation, irritability, or anger associated with it. The case presented below however was one of the most difficult I ever treated. There were many reasons for this, but the lack of patient compliance was the major problem. It also illustrates how to interpret very deep pulses as manifestations of emotions that are habitual or have been adapted to.

Sleep disorders are America's most frequent, deadliest, and costliest malady. A particular strength of the Chinese medical paradigm is that it gives an internal perspective on why insomnia develops. It is this precise differentiation that assists the practitioner in successful treatment. However, it is important to keep in mind that the emotions that accompany insomnia often make it difficult to cure. The patients are tired, frequently irritable, and sometimes desperate during their waking hours to get some rest.

The patient in this case was a fifty-seven-year-old female who had developed a sleeping disorder about four months previously. Her sleep pattern was characterized by an intense desire to go to bed early only to wake up three to five times during the night. She was clearly frantic.

Her insomnia was primarily of a deficient origin. In particular it was caused by a lack of the essential substances of qi and blood that were failing to anchor the spirit. Her variety of sleeplessness was also characterized by poor memory, lassitude, day-time drowsiness, dizziness, poor appetite, being easily frightened, shortness of breath, pallor, dry skin, and a stifling sensation in the chest. In addition, one of her arms twitched involuntarily. The pulse was deep and thready with an irregularity. The tongue, which was slightly purple with a red tip and almost no coat, was slightly deviated, wet, and quivery.

One year previously she had experienced an unidentified illness in which the symptoms were fever, swollen glands, and lethargy. She had worked extremely hard for a number of years (because it was necessary) and at that time her energy was "super." It had been a difficult time emotionally yet, "That is just the way it was," she reported. She clearly did not want to elaborate. About three years before seeing me she became noticeably colder, particularly in the evening. She lives in a very cold house in the mountains with no source of heat.

Her spirit needed to be treated—quieted and calmed—so that it would descend and become anchored in the material substrates of qi and blood. The problem was, of course, that qi and blood were inadequate and hence could not fulfill this function. The treatment strategy was a delicate balancing act of bringing the energy down from the head and rooting it, while simultaneously securing it by building qi and blood. To bring down the energy was rather easy, but to hold it there was difficult and lasted only temporarily because of the deficiency of qi and blood.

The patient demanded immediate and long-lasting results. Every successful step in treatment was a morsel, a promise of what was to come and the patient voraciously clamored for more. In addition, the patient did things that I thought could be exacerbating her condition. These activities included inversion therapy, hypnosis, hot baths before bed, sleeping on a magnetic bed, cranial-sacral therapy, elixir drinks, sleeping pills, and bizarre "blood purification" techniques. Because the patient moved from therapy to therapy, it was impossible to determine the effects of the therapies, positive or negative, if there were any at all.

The patient responded very well to acupuncture and moderately well to Chinese herbs. She always slept very well after a treatment. This pattern continued to improve for several months, but the results would only last for a few days at a time. More frequent visits were indicated, but were limited because the patient lived quite a distance away and was very conservative with her money.

After two months, the pulse, which had been so thin, but more importantly too deep, began to rise. There was a palpable Kidney pulse and the pulse in general was rising to the level appropriate for that time of year. At this point, I requested that the patient undergo some Western medical tests to refine the diagnosis. Even though significant improvement had been made in a short time with very little treatment, the patient was more dissatisfied and difficult to work with than ever. Her dalliance with other therapies made it hard for me to achieve stability in her case. There were other factors, such as hysteria, personal onslaughts on me as to why she could not sleep better, and the need to travel to my office that complicated the case. Also, she refused to see a Western physician because she was sure a medical condition would be discovered that her insurance company would not cover. All this set up the dynamics for a therapeutic relationship that reached an impasse.

This case presents several different lessons, not the least of which is to do the best we can and not become too attached to the outcome (which is not controlled by the practitioner anyway). But looking at the pathology, it was obvious that this patient's difficulties, supported by numerous signs and symptoms, centered around the Heart, its willingness to give, to receive, to laugh, to rest, to harmonize with the social world. The deep weak pulses indicated that her problem was related to the internal organs and to the yin organs in particular. It was a chronic problem that had been adapted to. As the recuperative energy of the body was tapped and strengthened, the pulse became stronger and higher. The emotions, even if in the form of complaints, began to surface, to be expressed, instead of being buried at the deep, hidden, adaptive level of the pulse. Now the patient needed to attend to her feelings. This remains the area that the patient needs to work on.

# CHAPTER 2

# THOUGHTS ON NEEDLING

The oldest Chinese medical text, the *Neijing (The Yellow Emperor's Classic),* provides timeless advice about needling. We must cultivate this knowledge before we have the privilege of inserting a needle into the human body to adjust the energy flow. The *Neijing* states, "The key to acupuncture lies in regulating the mind."[1] This statement from the *Neijing* has been explained by modern practitioners of Chinese medicine in China to mean that the accomplished acupuncturist must center the mind at the tip of the needle and at the acupuncture point to project his or her qi into the patient. Another dramatic quote from the *Neijing* admonishes, "Needling is like looking at a deep abyss; take care not to fall. . .Your hand must be like a hand grasping a tiger. One desires a kind of firm strength."[2]

Although ancient as well as modern practitioners recognize the legal and political implications of poor needle execution, this striking statement refers more to the seriousness and sacredness of misusing a needle in another person's body. Other quotes reinforce the profundity of wielding a needle and the importance of having a clear mind.

---

1. As quoted in Larée C and Rochat de la Vallee E: The practitioner-patient relationship: wisdom from the Chinese classics. *J Trad Acu,* Winter, 1990-91; 48.

2. The practitioner-patient relationship, 48.

"Know that you are on the edge of the mystery of life. Walk on the edge of the abyss without fear but have caution and circumspection not to fall. As a practitioner you must be deeply anchored and assured in your life. Yet the communication with the exterior passes through your orifices and your hand, which is holding the needle like a hand trying to hold a tiger. The tiger is the image of vital power."[3]

Anything healthcare practitioners do in their own lives to develop consciousness, attentiveness, and awareness will support their work as acupuncturists with intent. Whether it is gardening, calligraphy, painting, or housework, the goal is to bring full presence and attentiveness to the activity at hand. In the case of needling, we must possess the appropriate consciousness for this solemn task. If we regulate our breath by bringing it deep into the body through abdominal breathing, we help to regulate the mind and thus make our bodily energetics more rooted and secure. Finger strengthening exercises—such as the practice of inserting Chinese needles into an inch of newspapers without bending the needle *(see Figure 2, Needle Practice Pad)*—or opening the meridians of the arms by way of qi gong ball manipulations will strengthen the fingers and hands and regulate the mind so that we are prepared to execute the desired needle manipulations that will improve patient health. As the *Ode to the Explanation of Mysteries* reminds us, "If you should want to heal disease, there is nothing so

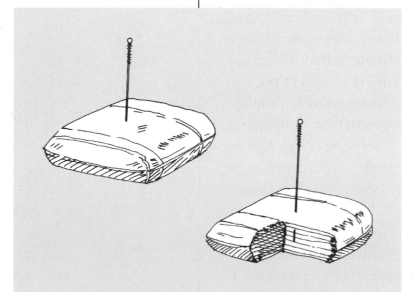

*Figure 2.* Needle Practice Pad

---

3. The practitioner-patient relationship, 48.

good as the needle."[4]  We must understand the profundity of using that needle.

Health is not simply a product of homeostasis initiated by inserting a needle.  It is a positive vision of a person ample in qi and blood, glowing with the vitality of the life force, whose materiality, spirit, and emotions are products of the upright qi of the body.  It is our responsibility as practitioners to possess this mindfulness, to visualize this possibility of human existence every time we treat a patient.  And acupuncture is not simply the insertion of a needle into the body which then automatically corrects its imbalances. The classics reinforce this fact when they state, "The unskilled physician grasps only the form when he uses the techniques of acupuncture. The superior physician understands the spirit."[5] We must safeguard the gift of life with the instrument of the needle.

This ancient understanding of the treatment of disease portrays human life as the integration of physical, emotional, and spiritual energies.  If we only adopt a material point of view when treating the human body, we will by definition not succeed.  If the patient's illness has not been cured, there are many variables that need to be reviewed, as I said in Chapter One.  For example, the practitioner must know whether to tonify or to sedate (disperse) and then make sure that the needle technique actually executed was indeed a tonification or a dispersion technique.  Even with all this, if the treatment is too materialistically oriented, too mechanistic, only the physical form, not the totality of the person's essence, will have been grasped.

Still, if we do not know how to manipulate the needle, the highest level of understanding of theory and the ability to turn theory into a diagnosis that captures the essence of the person is useless.

---

4. Dale RA:  Acupuncture needling: a summary of the principal traditional Chinese methods.  *Amer J Acupun,* 1994; 22(2): 167.

5. Acupuncture needling, 167.

# THE STAGES OF NEEDLING

**A**lthough the well-executed needle may seem to melt into the body in good Chinese technique or sink into the skin painlessly with a solid Japanese style, there are actually several integral steps to proficient needle technique that are not always apparent to the untrained eye because of the finesse of the skilled practitioner. These phases are delineated below.

## The Stages of Needling

### 1. Insertion, painless and sterile.

Insertion involves getting the needle into the skin (about fourteen layers of epidermis) in a sterile and painless manner. By "sterile" we mean that the shaft of the needle is not compromised by being touched with the bare hand or by an unsterile material such as gauze or cotton. For using Chinese needles, the classics prescribe, "The left hand is heavy and presses hard (on the point). This causes the qi to disperse. The right hand is light for entry and exit. In this way there is no pain."[1] Here, the acupuncturist is instructed in a two-handed needle technique where the point to be needled is pressed with one hand to stimulate the qi of the

---

1. From "Ode to the Standard of Mystery" as quoted in *Acupuncture, A Comprehensive Text,* Shanghai College of Traditional Chinese Medicine, Bensky D, O'Connor J (trans/eds). Eastland Press, Chicago, 1981; p 407.

channels and separate free nerve endings while the needle is inserted by the dominant hand with a thrust.

When using a tube with either a Chinese or Japanese needle, painless insertion can be achieved by firmly hitting the handle of the needle with the pads of the fingers as opposed to lightly tapping the head repeatedly. Common errors that acupuncturists who use needles with tubes often make, and that cause unnecessary pain to the patient, include the following:

1. Failing to disengage or detach the needle from the tube before attempting to tap it in.
2. Letting the needle tip sit too long on the skin.
3. Pushing it in inadvertently as it rests on the skin. Jing (well) and ear points, both located on thick skin, are good points to practice on when one has progressed beyond inserting a one-inch Chinese needle through a practice pad without bending the needle *(see Figure 2 in Chapter Two)*. Painless and sterile insertion is necessary to good needle technique and patient health.

## 2.  Going to the level of the qi.

Once the needle has been inserted without pain and in a sterile manner, it must now be pushed to the level of the qi, that is, where the qi resides. It is common knowledge that each point has a particular insertion depth that is determined by anatomical landmarks and meridian energetics. Underlying anatomical structures (vital organs, tendons, ligaments, major blood vessels, nerves, bone foramina, and so on) as well as individual variation in the patient's body size, sex, age, constitution, excesses, deficiencies, and the nature of the illness dictate where the qi will most likely be encountered. The practitioner's experience and treatment plan are also factors. No therapeutic result can be anticipated if the needle is not inserted to the level where the vital energy resides.

## 3. Getting the qi.

After the needle has been inserted to the level of the qi, the qi must now be contacted. As the Chinese claim, "getting the qi is half of the battle." This is the essence of needling. Without getting the qi, the treatment plan cannot proceed; that is, no subsequent tonification or dispersion can be initiated if the qi has not been engaged.

Techniques to get the qi are analogous to fishing. Teasing the energy in the body to the needle is like attracting a fish to the bait and the arrival of qi feels like a fish taking the line. Typically, the arrival of qi is signified by a feeling of tightness or fullness, like the manipulation of a needle in rubber. Common methods for getting the qi include but are not limited to the following, which are discussed below and summarized in *Table 2*.

### Lift and thrust.

Perpendicularly lift and thrust the needle but without too much force or the tissues may become damaged. This action coaxes the qi to the needle.

### Twirl.

Continuously rotate the needle back and forth, with small rotations in search of the qi. Never rotate the needle only in one direction as this action entwines the tissues and can cause pain.

### Retain the needle and wait.

A. Press along the meridian (following technique).

With the needle in place, press along the course of the meridian both above and below the needle to stimulate the vital qi, which may be weak.

B. Pluck.

Pluck the handle of the needle to cause a vibration to be conveyed along the course of the needle into the meridian. This method will smooth the qi along the channel in the event of any stagnation that is contributing to the slow arrival of the qi.

C.  Shake.

Shake the needle to strengthen the needle's presence, assist in the arrival of qi, and displace any perverse pathogen.

D.  Scrape.

Scrape the fingernail along the spiral head of a Chinese needle in an upward direction to bring the qi to the point.

E.  Rotate and release.

Use a "flying needle" technique.  This consists of rotating the needle in one direction until resistance is encountered and then suddenly releasing the needle.  Repeat this movement three times.  This method propagates and prolongs the needling sensation.

F.  Tremble.

In a movement termed the "trembling technique," use a simultaneous lift and thrust method with the twirling technique to attract the qi to the point.

G.  Needle a point nearby.

Needle a point nearby and along the course of the meridian to summon the qi to the point.

H.  Apply moxa.

Apply moxa to the affected area to promote the circulation of qi to the point.

Of course, in addition to manipulation methods, there are other factors that influence the arrival of qi to a point.  Some of the most important are correct point location, angle and depth of insertion, the age and constitution of the person, and the skill of the practitioner.

*Table 2.* Techniques for Getting the Qi

| |
|---|
| 1. Lift and thrust |
| 2. Twirl |
| 3. Retain and wait |

      a. Press along the course of the meridian
      b. Pluck the handle
      c. Shake the needle
      d. Scrape the handle
      e. Rotate and release
      f.  Simultaneously lift, thrust, and twirl
      g. Needle a point nearby
      h. Apply moxa

## 4. Manipulating the qi.

After the qi arrives *(da qi)*, something must be done with it. The engaged qi must be manipulated to achieve the therapeutic purpose of either strengthening and invigorating (tonifying) or sedating, draining, or breaking up (dispersing) the energy. The Chinese continue to remind us, "while half of the battle is getting the qi, the other half is what is done with it." Without attention to both these aspects of needling technique, the aim of the treatment will not be accomplished.

Although the Chinese treat most diseases with needle retention, the needle-retention time only strengthens and deepens the action of the technique. Conventional needle-retention times for tonification and sedation have been established, but in the final analysis, needles only have to be retained until the practitioner is sure that the goal of the treatment has been reached. There are other indications of therapeutic effectiveness that are more reliable than time. A change in pulse, patient demeanor, feeling the stimulus, a reaction to the stimulus, and also the skin's color can indicate that it is time to remove the needle. *Table 3,* although not comprehensive, summarizes some of the most common methods of tonifying and dispersing found in the literature and in clinical practice. Other techniques can be found in books about the treatment of disease as well as in the journal articles referenced below.[2] It is to the advantage of the patient that the practitioner be cognizant and proficient with as many techniques as possible so that the various patient experiences can best be treated.

*Table 3.* Concepts of Tonification and Sedation: Getting the Qi and Manipulating the Reaction

| | METHOD | |
|---|---|---|
| **VARIABLES** | **TONIFICATION** | **SEDATION** |
| Size of needles | Use thin needles | Use thick needles |
| Number of needles | Needle fewer points | Needle more points |
| Body type | For thin constitutional types | For heavier constitutional types |
| Condition | For chronic conditions | For acute conditions |
| When | Needle when the channel is weak (see channel's horary cycle time) | Needle when the channel is full (see channel's horary cycle time) |
| Moon | Needle at the new moon as the energy of the universe is increasing and supplementing | Needle at full moon, when the energy of the universe is full and the body needs to be drained |
| Depth | a. Needle superficially<br>b. Press the point heavily with the hand and insert the needle deeply | a. Needle deeply<br>b. Insert shallowly |
| Type of needles | Use gold or copper needles (yellow metals, which are yang) to strengthen | Use silver needles (white metals, which are yin) to cool |
| Other modalities | Use moxa, needles, exercise, diet, qi gong, rest, herbs | Use needles as the primary treatment modality |
| Type of points | Choose points that are tonification points or have tonifying energetics | Choose points that are sedation points or have sedation energetics |
| Direction and action relative to the meridian | a. Insert the needle in the direction of the meridian flow<br>b. For points of the Three Hand Yang and Three Foot Yin turn the needle clockwise<br>c. For points of the Three Hand Yin and Three Foot Yang turn the needle counter-clockwise | a. Insert the needle in the opposite direction to the meridian flow<br>b. For points of the Three Hand Yang and Three Foot Yin turn needle counter-clockwise<br>c. For points of the Three Hand Yin and Three Foot Yang turn the needle clockwise |
| Lift/thrust | Lift the needle slowly and gently, thrust heavily and rapidly | Lift the needle forcibly and rapidly, thrust gently and slowly |
| Amplitude and speed | Turn the needle with small amplitude (rotation) and slow speed | Turn the needle with large amplitude of rotation and fast speed |
| Sensation | Achieve no or a mild needling sensation | Achieve strong needling sensation |
| Time | Retain needles from 3–20 minutes. (Some sources say tonification should be longer than sedation) | Retain needles from 20 minutes to 1 hour. (Some sources say sedation should be shorter than tonification) |
| Insertion and withdrawal | a. Insert the needle slowly and withdraw quickly<br>b. Insert on the inhale, withdraw on exhale<br>c. Insert on the exhale, withdraw on inhale | a. Insert the needle quickly and withdraw slowly<br>b. Insert on the exhale, withdraw on inhale<br>c. Insert on the inhale, withdraw on exhale |
| Site | Apply pressure by closing the hole with clean, dry cotton immediately after taking the needle out | Enlarge the hole upon withdrawal by shaking the needle and leave the hole open |
| Direction | One large clockwise turn followed by three small counter-clockwise turns | Three small counter-clockwise turns followed by one large clockwise turn |
| Type of person | Shallow depth for more sensitive patients | Deep and strong for less sensitive patients |
| Condition | Deficiency | Excess |
| Frequency | Once - intermittent i.e., manipulate slightly (a few seconds), rest, repeat | Vigorously or continuously until symptoms are relieved (from several minutes to several hours as in the case of anesthesia) |
| Moxibustion | Apply more | Apply less |

*Notes: Tonification and sedation are always relative. Also this chart contains varied opinions about insertion and withdrawal.*

2. Dale RA: Acupuncture needling: a summary of the principal traditional Chinese methods. *Amer J Acupun*, 1994; 22(2): 167. See also Kudriavtsev A: Needling methods: translation and commentary on the Ode to tonification, sedation and a clear conscience *(Bu xie xu xin ge)* from the "Great Compendium of Acupuncture and Moxibustion" *(Zhen Jiu Da Chang)*. *Amer J Acupun*, 1992; 20(2): 143–150.

## 5. Withdrawal.

Needling is not complete until the needle has been removed. Needles should be carefully and nontraumatically removed. Force should never be used to disengage a needle from a point. If a needle appears to be stuck, it may have been inserted too forcefully or manipulated too vigorously and in the future the practitioner should be more careful. If the practitioner does experience such a situation when withdrawing the needle the following approaches can be tried:

1. Gently massage around another point close by to attract the qi from the stuck needle.
2. Needle another point in close proximity for similar reasons, and
3. If the needle seems to be entwined in the tissue, try to turn it slowly in the opposite direction to disengage it.

## 6. Dealing with the site.

The final stage of needling, following withdrawal of the needle, concerns the needle site. *Table 3* also summarizes

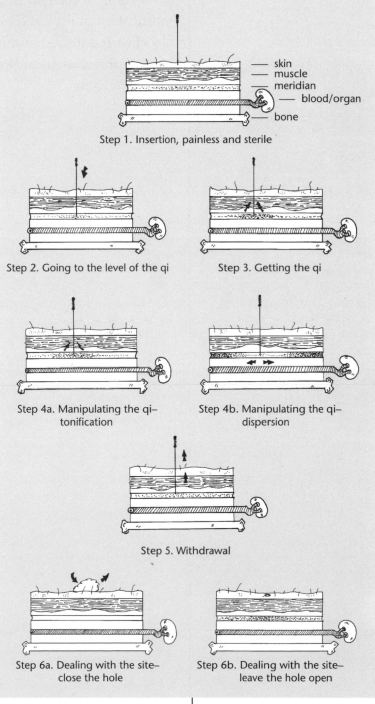

Step 1. Insertion, painless and sterile

— skin
— muscle
— meridian
— blood/organ
— bone

Step 2. Going to the level of the qi

Step 3. Getting the qi

Step 4a. Manipulating the qi–
tonification

Step 4b. Manipulating the qi–
dispersion

Step 5. Withdrawal

Step 6a. Dealing with the site–
close the hole

Step 6b. Dealing with the site–
leave the hole open

*Figure 3.* The Stages of Needling

commonly accepted notions of what to do with the puncture site after needling (that is, close the hole for tonification or leave it open for dispersion).  In the event of bleeding or ecchymosis, the practitioner, regardless of tonification or dispersion technique, should absorb the blood with a sterile cotton ball and apply pressure to the bruised or tender area.  *Figure 3* shows the stages of needling in graphic form.

# WHAT IS A POINT?

The classics remind us that the aim of the five branches of Oriental healing therapy is to establish a connection between the patient, and to effect a change,[1] whether that change be through acupuncture, herbs, massage, nutrition, or exercise/breathing therapy.  In acupuncture, where the tool for this connection is the needle, correct needle technique—as well as precise point location and astute point selection—is the prerequisite to achieving the desired therapeutic result.

The energetics or functions of the points are numerous and essentially correspond to the physiological functions of the body.  The clinical experience of Chinese medicine seems to suggest that the points are capable of correcting the physiological deficiencies that humans are prone to unless the vital qi is so diminished or deranged that the balance cannot be redressed. Because of the proliferation of point functions that have been developed over the years, the beginning student or novice practitioner of Oriental medicine often become lost in the many point functions.  They struggle to see some rhyme or reason why each point possesses the roles that as students they had to routinely memorize.

If one thing can be said about Oriental medicine

---

1.  Larée C and Rochat de la Vallee E: The patient-practitioner relationship: wisdom from the Chinese classics. *J Trad Acu,* Winter, 1990-91; 14.

(apart from its effectiveness as shown through the centuries), it is that it is an inherently logical medicine. That is not to say that there are no inconsistencies within its vast body of experience, for there are. (These inconsistencies may actually be a source of strength to the system because of the options they present.) However, the Chinese medical system is logical in the sense that pathology can be predicted if physiology is understood; diagnosis dictates treatment principles; and point energetics are a product of the classical, physiological roles those points play in the organism.

The role of points in the human body can be viewed from a variety of perspectives. The Chinese remind us that in discussing the identity of acupuncture points, both the anatomic and physiologic aspects need to be considered. That is, where the point is and what the point does are contributing factors to understanding the energetics of points. The way I like to think about the points, which concurs with this Chinese assessment, is that where a point "lives" (its location) and what a point does (its function) are akin to a "job description" that contributes to its unique identity.

A survey of the acupuncture literature offers further insight into the question, "what is a point?" Etymologically, the word for point, *xue*, denotes a cave or hole. This translation suggests how the Chinese viewed this site. The word also evokes the notion that demons, especially wind demons, could live in these holes, either in nature or in the body. Over time, this hole came to connote a place where qi was able to penetrate the body as well as flow out.[2] The Chinese character for "hole" was combined with the character for "passage, transport, and qi" so that the point came to be perceived as a route to the interior. As such, the points were channels of communication between the external and internal environments. Pathogens could enter the

---

2. Unschuld P: *Medicine in China, A History of Ideas.* University of California Press, Berkeley, 1985; p 71.

body here.[3]  The *Spiritual Axis* claimed, "points are places where the qi roams in and out."[4]

Classically, the points were viewed as anatomical locations on the body where the qi and blood could be accessed.  Points were seen as sites where the qi of the zang-fu organs and channels is transported to the body surface.  Because there are relative excesses and deficiencies in the body, the points were considered as places where these imbalances could be approached and changed.  When the human body is affected by disease, we can treat the patient by puncturing points on the surface of the body to regulate the qi and blood of the channels.  The image of the point as a hole or a gate that allows the entry and exit of qi provides a living, functional image of the point as an active physiological nexus instead of as a static, anatomical location.

So, for example, if we want to bring energy to the point, we "tonify" it;  if we want to take energy away from an area through the point, we "disperse" (sedate) it.  The various ways of accomplishing these two basic movements of energy are listed in *Table 3*, found in Chapter Three.

There are further anatomical analogies that support the model of a point as a working physiological location that can reflect the point's job description.  Historically, one definition of points included areas that had different consistencies, discolorations, or were more moist or dry than surrounding areas.[5]  This description points to the importance of cultivating perception through inspection and palpation by the practitioner, thus assisting not only point location but diagnosis as well.  Other findings that support the contention that points reflect the "physiology gone wrong" can be found in *Table 4*.

---

3. Van Nghi N: Luo point use in traditional Chinese medicine.  Lecture,  Southwest Acupuncture College, Santa Fe, N.M., Sept., 1986.

4. As quoted in *Acupuncture, A Comprehensive Text*, Shanghai College of Traditional Chinese Medicine, Bensky D, O'Connor J (trans/eds).  Eastland Press, Chicago, 1981: p 401.

5. *Acupuncture*, p 40.

*Table 4.* Signs of Point Pathology:  Derived from the Five
Methods of Diagnosis

| A. INSPECTION (Things that can be Seen) | B. AUSCULTATION (Heard) | C. OLFACTION (Smelled) | D. PALPATION (Felt) | E. INQUIRY (Asked About) |
|---|---|---|---|---|
| rashes | gurgling (fluid accumulation sounds) | Five Element smells: | Pain: | All of the pathology related to the Five Preliminaries and the Ten Questions |
| moles | | scorched | referred | |
| warts | | fragrant | sharp, fixed | |
| petechiae | inhalations and exhalations | rotten | stabbing | |
| depressions | | putrid | boring | |
| asymmetries | sounds, sighs, and so on | rancid | dull | |
| boils | | | awareness | |
| lumps | | | consciousness | |
| lesions | | | burning | |
| varicosities | | | hot | |
| scars | | | movement to a particular place deep, superficial | |
| bruises | | | | |
| swellings, edema, puffiness, bloating | | | gummy | |
| redness | | | knots | |
| bone growths | | | pulsations | |
| dryness/wetness | | | visible tension | |
| inversions/eversions | | | mushiness | |
| knots | | | softness | |
| hair presence or absence | | | lack of tone | |
| buffalo humps | | | hard like a rock or a stone | |
| fat (overweight) | | | cold | |
| leanness/gauntness | | | dry | |
| leathery | | | wet | |
| withered | | | chopstick hardness | |
| prolapses | | | | |
| growths | | | | |
| size of the sternocostal angle | | | | |
| pulsations | | | | |
| depth of the breathing | | | | |
| shoulder posture | | | | |
| muscle bands | | | | |
| flushing colorations | | | | |
| birthmarks | | | | |
| hairy patches | | | | |

*Since the focus of this book is not diagnostic, the clinical significance of each of these diagnostic findings can be pursued in basic texts, differentiation-of-disease books, and in my forthcoming book, "The Magic Hand Returns Spring, The Art of Palpatory Diagnosis."*

The *Neijing* posits a maxim that most acupuncturists are well aware of, that is, "where there is a painful spot, there is an acupuncture point." The significance of this statement is that pain or discomfort from either excess or deficiency represents pathology in the body. Sometimes such pain is overt, that is, the patient is aware of it and articulates it either as a major complaint or as part of the internal landscape. Other times though, pain is below the threshold of consciousness and can only be significantly evoked and grappled with when the body is palpated.

We must remember that one of the methods of traditional diagnosis is palpation. Because of time constraints in a student clinic setting, and even in major hospitals in China, palpation has in my opinion become an almost lost art. While it is not the purpose of this book to summarize all the advantages of palpation that elevate it to the most subtle and sublime of diagnostic arts, it is still important to point out that precise point location can often be ascertained through inspection and palpation of suspect areas.

Acupuncture, the needling of points on the human body for the purpose of adjusting the flow of energy, is a means of affecting what goes on inside the body because it influences the activity of the substances moving through the meridians. As Ted Kaptchuck so eloquently and aptly summarized, stimulating points can reduce what is excessive, increase what is deficient, warm what is cold, cool what is hot, circulate what is stagnant, move what is congealed, stabilize what is reckless, raise what is falling, and lower what is rising.[6]

In short, considering the Chinese outlook, a point can be viewed as an anatomical location through which exogenous pathogens can enter and be dispersed or through which the physiological function of the human body can be regulated and stimulated *(see Figure 4).*

---

6. Kaptchuck T: *The Web That Has No Weaver.* Congdon and Weed, New York, 1983; pp 79–80.

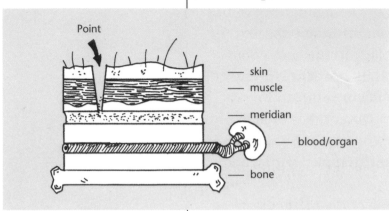

***Figure 4.*** What is a Point?

Although anatomical descriptions are meaningful road maps that can denote the general area of the point, a point must be thought of as three dimensional. Points are distinguished partly by their surface anatomical landmarks, but they also possess an underlying anatomy that can consist of organs, innervations, and vascularizations. As the *Inner Classic* states, "the twelve channels circulate deep within the muscle and cannot be seen."[7]

For different points, qi resides at different depths. The functional capacity of a point is partly derived from its depth—and likewise qi converges at different depths because of its function. To access the qi and stimulate the appropriate point function, the correct needle technique, that is, the angle and depth of insertion for the particular point, is imperative.

Seasoned practitioners know that accurate point location is not a function of mathematical calculations done on the body. Rather, because the point incarnates a living energy, a point, embedded as it is in connective tissue, could be more accurately viewed as energy in motion. Also, people vary anatomically. For instance, one may lack the tendon of the muscle palmaris longus, another may have six lumbar vertebrae or an attached eleventh rib, or scars over points, and so on. In these cases, the anatomical description of a point can only get the practitioner to the general area of the point. Palpation and inspection are unparalleled tools for the practitioner, not only in these anomalous cases but for all correct point location.

Western scientists, intrigued with Oriental medicine, are not without their theories on what a point is

7. *Acupuncture*, p 111.

and they have advanced a number of propositions.[8] It is common knowledge in the scientific community that points can be electrically located, and they are considered part of the electromagnetic field of the body. It has been determined that this field is not uniformly dense. Where decreased electrical resistance and increased electrical conductivity are detected, the areas correspond to acupuncture points whose functions are deficient. Where an increase in ionic concentration is indicated by increased electrical resistance, the corresponding point function may be pathological in the Chinese sense as well, that is, there may be excess conditions such as stagnation, presence of pathogens, and so on. These are the mechanisms whereby electropoint detectors work. According to the Zhang-Popp hypothesis, treatment by acupuncture needling causes a disturbance in the standard wave pattern caused by a new boundary. Changes in the electrical potential because of wounding (like that produced by needling) have been investigated by Robert Becker and others. "Currents of injury result such that the needled region becomes a new EM [electromagnetic] field source with concomitant interference effects over the whole body."[9]

Using the circulatory systems as the explanation for how a point works was dismissed early on because the blood and lymph flows lacked the speed with which the stimulation of a point could affect tissues and other functions. On the other hand, nervous system involvement has been investigated and there seems to be a strong, though by no means comprehensive, correlation between this regulatory system and how acupuncture works.

In 1959, researchers at the Shanghai College of Traditional Medicine noted that there is a close rela-

8. Rubik B: Can western science provide a foundation for acupuncture? *Alt Ther,* Sept., 1995; (1)4.

9. Western science, 45.

tionship between peripheral nerves in the tissues and the acupuncture points. Of the 309 points studied, 152 points stimulated were over nerves and seventy-three were close by—within .5 centimeters. In 1969, they noted that 323 points were directly supplied by nerves, 304 were supplied by superficial cutaneous nerves, 155 by deeper nerves, and 137 had both deep and superficial involvement. From dissections and observation under microscopes, it was determined that all layers of the skin and muscle tissues at the acupuncture sites contained numerous and varied nerve endings.

Additionally, it was observed that points congregated close to nerves and consequently could be located in predictable places. The larger the peripheral nerve, especially those identifiable in gross anatomy, the more likely they were to have points distributed along them. The depth of the peripheral nerve was also an important variable. As peripheral nerves emerge from deep to superficial, points are likely to form along their nerve routes. Points could also be found where nerves penetrate the deep fascia, where a nerve emerges from a bone foramina, where a muscular branch of a peripheral nerve attaches and enters a muscle mass, and at the bifurcation point of peripheral nerves. Likewise, blood vessels were frequently seen in the vicinity of neuromuscular attachments.[10]

Further implication of the nervous system in the action of points is found in the viscero-cutaneous theory. According to this perspective, internal diseases of the organs produce pain or tenderness at certain acupuncture points or in areas of the skin known as dermatomes. This idea corresponds with Felix Mann's notion of the generalized site: an internal organ can become so sensitive that it can refer to a larger-than-normal skin area.

Although these observations represent important contributions by the modern scientific community

10. *Acupuncture*, p 111.

about how acupuncture points may work, it is evident that these theories cannot explain the richness of point function that is part of the repertoire of Chinese medicine. On the other hand, the classical Chinese physicians have offered us an elegant and economical framework for organizing points. They have not only helped us to comprehend and predict point function, but they also have described mechanisms internally consistent with their theories of organ physiology, essential substances, and the etiology of disease. Their point classification system is discussed in the next chapter.

5

# THE POINT CLASSIFICATION SYSTEM

Like stars in the constellations, the acupuncture points are distributed over the body along the energy pathways known as meridians. The vital energy of the body infuses these points. As the classics explain, without qi and blood there is no place in the human body that can be living and healthy.[1]

In answer to the question "How many points are there?" the Chinese respond, "As many as there are painful places." However, it is important to note that these painful places are not only spots where the spontaneous firing of nerves occurs, but also locations where there is tenderness on palpation or with other mechanical stimulation. (For a discussion of the functional phases of points, that is, the health of a point, see Chapter Fourteen).

The initial classification of points begins with organizing all the points of the human body into three major categories: the Extraordinary points, the *ah shi* points, and the points of the fourteen channels.

## The Extraordinary Points

The Extraordinary points, also known as the Nonmeridian points, are points that have definite

---

1. Weisman N and Ellis A: *Fundamentals of Chinese Medicine.* Paradigm Publications, Brookline, Mass., 1985; p 23.

locations and known energetics but that are not located along the course of a meridian. Sometimes they are referred to as Experiential or Clinically Effective points. They number in the hundreds and are specified by name or number, for example, Taiyang or M-HN-9.[2] Functionally, they are useful points to supplement the points of the fourteen channels.

## The Ah Shi Points

The ah shi points (tender, "Oh, yes!" points) are those that either fire spontaneously or are discovered by palpation or other mechanical means. Their number is virtually unlimited. They do not have definite locations or names.

## The Points of the Fourteen Channels

The points of the fourteen channels, also known as the regular points, have specific locations and actions. There are 361 of them along the meridians. *Table 5* lists the number of points located on each channel.

*Table 5.* Points of the Fourteen Channels

| MERIDIAN | STANDARD NOMENCLATURE OF MERIDIAN* | NUMBER OF POINTS |
|---|---|---|
| Lung | LU | 11 |
| Large Intestine | LI | 20 |
| Stomach | ST | 45 |
| Spleen | SP | 21 |
| Heart | HT | 9 |
| Small Intestine | SI | 19 |
| Bladder | BL | 67 |
| Kidney | KI | 27 |
| Pericardium | PC | 9 |
| Triple Warmer | TE | 23 |
| Gall Bladder | GB | 44 |
| Liver | LR | 14 |
| Governing Vessel | GV | 28 |
| Conception Vessel | CV | 24 |

*Standard nomenclature by the World Health Organization, 1989.*

2. Shanghai College of Traditional Chinese Medicine: *Acupuncture, A Comprehensive Text.* Bensky D, O' Connor J (trans/eds). Eastland Press, Chicago, 1981; p 145.

The points of the fourteen channels can be further arranged into ten major categories that are useful in appreciating their functional roles in the body. The clinical significance of each group is discussed below.

## A. Yuan (Source) points

Each of the twelve main meridians has a yuan (source) point located bilaterally on the extremities. As the name implies, they are points where the original qi, our inherited essence, is stored or pooled. They are very effective points for both diagnosis and treatment because of this property.

The yuan points stimulate the vital energy of the twelve main meridians, regulate the functional activities of the internal organs, reinforce the antipathogenic factor, and eliminate pathogenic causes of disease. They are useful points for treating the root of a problem, particularly disorders of the internal organs. They are generally used for chronic problems.

The Source point of a meridian has a strong relationship to the Luo point of its coupled meridian. Because of this relationship, the coupled meridian's Luo point can tap into some of this consigned essence. (See Chapter Six for clinical strategies on how to use Luo points.)

Just as the jing (well) point and the ying (spring) point are always the first and second-most distal points on a meridian respectively, the Source point is invariably the third-most distal point on a yin meridian. LU 9 (Taiyuan), HT 7 (Shenmen), and SP 3 (Taibai) are examples of this rule. On a yin meridian the shu (stream) point and the Source point are the same, thus making these points more potent.

On a yang meridian, the fourth-most distal point with the exception of the Gall Bladder meridian is always the source point. Thus, LI 4 (Hegu), SI 4 (Wangu), and BL 64 (Jinggu) are Source points.

## B.  Luo (Connecting) Points

Each of the twelve main meridians possesses a Luo point.  In addition, the Conception and the Governing Vessels each have one and the Spleen has two, its regular Luo point and one known as the Grand Luo.  Some sources claim that ST 18 (Rugen) is also a Luo point that connects the Stomach to the Heart.[3]

Luo points can be used in two ways, either as transverse or longitudinal vessels.  In treatment, the way to differentiate a longitudinal from a transverse Luo is by the angle of insertion of the needle.  Therefore, the importance of correct needle technique cannot be overestimated for achieving the desired therapeutic result.

A transverse Luo sends a stimulus directly to the Source point of its coupled organ.  For instance, when we stimulate LI 6 (Pianli), the Luo point of the Large Intestine meridian, it sends energy to its coupled source point, LU 9 (Taiyuan).  This technique links the internal-external meridians together, that is, it connects the coupled organ-meridian complexes in the Five Element system.  The effect of such a treatment plan is to create a homeostatic connection between the two coupled meridians so that, for example, Large Intestine energy can be tapped and brought to the Lung meridian.

A longitudinal Luo links with its corresponding organ, and stimulates that organ.  In the same way, when it is needled longitudinally, LI 6 (Pianli) sends a stimulus to the Large Intestine *organ* itself.  In this case, the Large Intestine *meridian* is stimulated directly instead of Large Intestine energy being borrowed to stimulate Lung function as in the previous illustration.

There are other Luos that do not connect yin/yang couples together, such as the *Bao luo*, a special communication vessel between the Kidney and the uterus; the Luo of the Ren channel, which connects to the abdo-

---

3. *Acupuncture*, p 36.

men and dominates the collaterals of the yin channels; the Luo of the Governing Vessel channel, which goes to the head and dominates the collaterals of the yin channels; and the Grand Luo of the Spleen, which goes to the hypochondriac region and connects all the Luo points as well as the blood vessels. In addition, there are four group Luos: SP 6 (Sanyinjiao), the group Luo of the Three Leg Yin; GB 39 (Xuanzhong), group Luo of the Three Leg Yang; PC 5 (Jianshi), group Luo of the Three Arm Yin; and TE 8 (Sanyangluo), group Luo of the Three Arm Yang. These group Luos, because of their multiple intersections, are strong points for activating the energy of the meridians they control. Chapter Six fully explains and includes various opinions on the use of Luo points both theoretically and practically with the correct needle technique.

## C. Xi (cleft) points.

There are sixteen Xi (cleft) points: one from each of the twelve main meridians and four from certain Curious Vessels. As the name implies, Xi (cleft) points occur where the qi of the channel is deeply converged in a cleft. A perusal of the insertion depths for acupuncture points along a meridian shows that typically they are slightly deeper for a Xi (cleft) point than for adjacent points along the same meridian [see *Figure 5*, Location of Xi (cleft) Points].

*Figure 5.* Location of Xi (cleft) Points

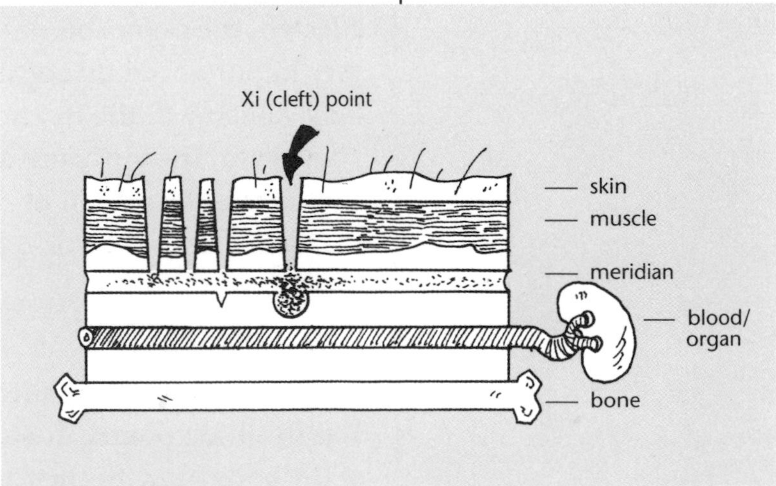

Xi (cleft) points are all located on the extremities (i.e. below the knees or above the elbow) with the exception of ST 34 (Liangqiu), the only Xi (cleft) point located above the knees. Xi (cleft) points are considered to be meridian reflex points, meaning that they show the health of a meridian. When palpated or observed for abnormal colorations they can be used as diagnostic points of the meridians. Xi (cleft) points are utilized for acute disorders that manifest as pain, accumulation, stagnation, and inflammation in an area. For instance, ST 34 (Liangqiu) is beneficial for stomachache and SP 8 (Diji) for menstrual cramps. Xi (cleft) points can be used for any inflammation. This usage is certainly not an insignificant energetic.

## D.  Front Mu points

Front Mu points, also known as Alarm points or Front Collecting points, are of the utmost clinical significance in the point classification system. There are twelve Front Mu points all located on the chest and abdomen, each related to one of the twelve main meridians.

Because the Front Mu points are close to their respective organs, it is not surprising that the qi (yin and yang bound together) of the zang-fu is infused in these points. They are particularly reactive to pathological changes in the body and when the organs are affected, the points become tender. Front Mu points, very important in diagnosis and treatment, are particularly valuable in the treatment of chronic disorders. They reveal the yin/yang disharmony of each organ and, as the classics tell us, when the six fu are diseased, the yang diseases devolve to their yin aspect.

## E.  Back Shu points

Back Shu points, also called Associated points or Back Transforming points, are located on the ventral surface of the body close to their respective organs and parallel to the vertebral column. The qi and blood of the organs are infused in the Back Shu points, thus they are particularly helpful in distinguishing qi and blood pathology. The Front Mu points, in contrast, are better for discriminating yin and yang disharmonies.

There are twelve pairs of Back Shu points, one pair for each of the twelve zang-fu organs, and also for a number of other organs and structures—for instance the diaphragm and the lumbar vertebrae. *Table 6* lists the Front Mu and Back Shu points of the twelve main meridians, the organs, and structures.

*Table 6.* Front Mu and Back Shu Points

| MERIDIAN/ORGAN/STRUCTURE | FRONT MU | BACK SHU |
| --- | --- | --- |
| Lung | LU 1 | BL 13 |
| Large Intestine | ST 25 | BL 25 |
| Stomach | CV 12 | BL 21 |
| Spleen | LR 13 | BL 20 |
| Heart | CV 15 | BL 15 |
| Small Intestine | CV 4 | BL 27 |
| Bladder | CV 3 | BL 28 |
| Kidney | GB 25 | BL 23 |
| Pericardium | CV 17 | BL 14 |
| Triple Warmer | CV 5 | BL 22 |
| Gall Bladder | GB 24 | BL 19 |
| Liver | LR 14 | BL 18 |
| Governing Vessel | X | BL 16 |
| Conception Vessel | X | X |
| Bones | X | BL 11 |
| Upper Lung | X | BL 12 |
| Diaphragm | X | BL 17 |
| Lumbar Vertebrae | X | BL 24 |
| Lower Lumbar | X | BL 26 |
| Sacrum | X | BL 29 |
| Bladder sphincter | X | BL 30 |

X = None

## F.  Influential points

The Eight Influential points are a noteworthy group of points that exert special influence on their associated entities.  Additionally, these points have other important energetics that further enhance their status.  The Eight Influential points and what they dominate are listed in *Table 7*.

*Table 7.* The Eight Influential Points

| POINT | AREA OF INFLUENCE | POINT | AREA OF INFLUENCE |
|---|---|---|---|
| LR 13 | Zang organs | LU 9 | Vessels |
| CV 12 | Fu organs | GB 39 | Marrow |
| BL 17 | Blood | CV 17 | Qi |
| GB 34 | Tendons | BL 11 | Bone |

## G. Confluent points

The Eight Confluent points, also known as Master points, refer to the points of each of the Eight Curious Vessels that activate the physiology pertaining to those vessels. In addition, each Curious Vessel also has a Coupled point, that is, a point that when activated, works well with its corresponding meridian. Although certain Curious Vessels operate well in pairs, they can also be used separately to treat disorders of the corresponding meridian (see Chapter Eleven on the use of the Eight Curious Vessels in general). The Confluent points are strong points for treatment because of their connection with the Eight Curious Vessels in addition to the fact that these points also control other significant energetics. *Table 8* below lists the Eight Curious Vessels along with their Master and Coupled points.

*Table 8.* The Master and Coupled Points of the Eight Curious Vessels

| MERIDIAN | MASTER POINT | COUPLED POINT |
|---|---|---|
| Du | SI 3 | BL 62 |
| Ren | LU 7 | KI 6 |
| Chong | SP 4 | PC 6 |
| Dai | GB 41 | TE 5 |
| Yinqiao | KI 6 | LU 7 |
| Yangqiao | BL 62 | SI 3 |
| Yinwei | PC 6 | SP 4 |
| Yangwei | TE 5 | GB 41 |

## H. Coalescent points

Coalescent points are defined as intersection points between the Eight Curious Vessels and the twelve main meridians. As has been obvious throughout this discussion, the greater the range of energetics of a point, the greater its clinical utility. Examples of coalescent points include BL 1 (Jingming), the intersection of the Bladder and Yangqiao meridians; GB 20 (Fengchi), the intersection of the Gall Bladder, Yangwei, and Yangqiao meridians; and ST 8 (Touwei), intersection of the Stomach and Yangwei meridians. Other Coalescent points can be found in most standard texts.

## I. Crossing points

Crossing points, also referred to as Union points or points of reunion, represent points of intersection between two or more main channels. Most of these ninety points are located on the head, face, and trunk. They are very efficient points to use because of their multiple intersections. Examples of important crossing points include CV 3 (Zhongji), meeting of the Three Leg Yin on the abdomen, and ST 13 (Qihu), meeting of the Stomach, Large Intestine, and Triple Burner meridians. Other crossing points can be found in most standard point books.

## J. The Five Shu points

The Five Shu points, also referred to as the Five Command or Antique points, are a particular collection of points on the twelve main meridians that are located between the elbow and fingertips on the upper limbs and on the knee and toe tips on the lower extremities. The energy in these five special points is like the energy found in different bodies of water from a well to a sea. Similarly, qi flows in the meridians like water and builds up force and depth as it flows from distal to proximal vortices.

Each of the twelve main meridians has five Shu points, and regardless of the meridian, each Shu point has certain therapeutic properties in common that indicate how to use that cluster of points.

Tables *9, 10,* and *11* are practical charts that outline the Five Shu points in terms of their analogy to a body of water, that is, the amount of qi they contain. *Table 9* illustrates the point number on a meridian; indicates the element point they are on the meridian; describes the action of each type of point; and lists common clinical conditions for which each type of point can be used.

**Table 9.** The Use of the Command Points for the Amount of Qi They Contain

| SHU POINT | POINTS ON MERIDIAN (Distal to Proximal) | YIN MERIDIAN | YANG MERIDIAN | ENERGY OF THE POINT | CLINICAL CONDITIONS |
|---|---|---|---|---|---|
| Jing (well) | #1 on tips of extremities (sides of nails or tips of fingers and toes) | Wood | Metal | The qi of the channel starts to bubble. The meridian's energy bubbles, exchanging energy to effect a change in polarity. The point stimulates the meridian as well as the tendinomuscular meridian. | Sore throat, apoplexy, toothache, coma, chest fullness, mental diseases related to zang organs |
| Ying (spring) | #2 | Fire | Water | The qi of the channels starts to gush; water has just started to trickle from a spring. | Febrile disease |
| Shu (stream) | #3 | Earth | Wood | The qi of the channel flourishes, like a stream with stronger movement. | Joint pain caused by pathogenic heat and damp, heavy sensation of the body |
| Jing (river) | Not able to be consistently numbered | Metal | Fire | The qi of the channel increases in abundance, pouring abundantly. There is much more flow, like the water on which boats can travel. | Asthma, throat, cough disorders |
| He (sea) | Elbow or knee | Water | Earth | The qi of the channel is the most flourishing. There are large amounts of energy going deeper. | Intestinal or digestive problems, diarrhea, six fu organ diseases, diseases of the stomach and intestine |

*Table 10* specifically illustrates a classical method of using the Five Shu points in treating various levels of attack.

*Table 10.* The Use of the Command Points for the Level of Attack

| SHU POINT | JING (well) | YING (spring) | SHU (stream) | JING (river) | HE (sea) |
|---|---|---|---|---|---|
| Seasonal usage | The season of spring, as well as the *spring* of a disease | Summer, the *summer* of a disease | Late summer, the *late summer* of a disease | Fall, the *fall* of a disease | Winter, the *winter* of a disease |
| Clinical Manifestations | Mental disorders, chest disorders, coma, unconsciousness, stifling sensation in chest, acute problems, apparent fullness, first aid, yin organ problems | Fevers, febrile diseases | Painful joints caused by pathogenic heat and damp, yin organ problems | Asthma, throat, cough disorders, alternating chills and fever, muscle and bone problems | Disorders of the fu organs, bleeding stomach, diarrhea, (tends not to affect the meridian at this level) |

*Table 11* details the acupuncture points that correspond to the Five Shu points. As is obvious from the chart, if we know the number of points on a meridian and where the meridian begins and ends, we can determine the jing (well), ying (spring), shu (stream), and yuan (source) points without memorizing them.

The Five Shu points are popular, especially with classically trained practitioners, whether they be Chinese, Japanese, or Korean. They are very effective points of treatment as their energetics suggest. There is sometimes an unpleasant needling sensation felt at the most distal points, but good needle technique at these locations can substantially reduce this. In addition, immense therapeutic advantages can generally only be achieved with these points.

The previous discussion of the Five Shu points has

*Table 11.* Acupuncture Points that Correspond to the Five Shu Points

| MERIDIAN | JING (well) | YING (spring) | SHU (stream) | YUAN (source) | JING (river) | HE (sea) | LUO | XI (cleft) | LOWER HE (sea) | UPPER HE (sea) |
|---|---|---|---|---|---|---|---|---|---|---|
| LU | 11 | 10 | 9 | 9 | 8 | 5 | 7 | 6 | X | X |
| LI | 1 | 2 | 3 | 4 | 5 | 11 | 6 | 7 | ST 37 | LI 9 |
| SP | 1 | 2 | 3 | 3 | 5 | 9 | 4 | 8 | X | X |
| ST | 45 | 44 | 43 | 42 | 41 | 36 | 40 | 34 | X | LI 10 |
| HT | 9 | 8 | 7 | 7 | 4 | 3 | 5 | 6 | X | X |
| SI | 1 | 2 | 3 | 4 | 5 | 8 | 7 | 6 | ST 39 | LI 8 |
| BL | 67 | 66 | 65 | 64 | 60 | 40 | 58 | 63 | X | X |
| KI | 1 | 2 | 3 | 3 | 7 | 10 | 4 | 5 | X | X |
| PC | 9 | 8 | 7 | 7 | 5 | 3 | 6 | 4 | X | X |
| TE | 1 | 2 | 3 | 4 | 6 | 10 | 5 | 7 | BL 39 | X |
| GB | 44 | 43 | 41 | 40 | 38 | 34 | 37 | 36 | X | X |
| LR | 1 | 2 | 3 | 3 | 4 | 8 | 5 | 6 | X | X |
| GV | X | X | X | X | X | X | 1 | X | X | X |
| CV | X | X | X | X | X | X | 15 | X | X | X |
| Yinqiao | X | X | X | X | X | X | X | KI 8 | X | X |
| Yang-qiao | X | X | X | X | X | X | X | BL 59 | X | X |
| Yinwei | X | X | X | X | X | X | X | KI 9 | X | X |
| Yangwei | X | X | X | X | X | X | X | GB 35 | X | X |

*X = no point*

*Lower He (sea): The three yang meridians of the hand (the Large Intestine, the Small Intestine, and the Triple Warmer) are represented on the foot on another yang meridian.*

outlined how to classify these points of the human body into categories based on general energetics. These categories can help us understand the nature of a particular point, but there is also an additional property. They also carry an elemental energy related to the Five Elements and this energy confers upon the point its rudimentary value.

As is well known by practitioners, the most distal Shu point on a yin meridian is always a wood point followed by fire, earth, metal, and water in the order of the five elements. For instance on the Lung meridian, LU 11 (Shaoshang), the jing (well) point and the most distal Shu point, is the wood point. LU 10 (Yuji), the ying (spring) point, is the fire point; LU 9 (Taiyuan), the shu (stream) point, is the earth point; LU 8 (Jingqu), the jing (river) point, is the metal point; and finally, LU 5 (Chize), the he (sea) point, is the water point.

On a yang meridian, the most distal Shu point is

always a metal point. Correspondingly, the rest of the distal Shu points have water, wood, fire, and earth energy assigned to them, in that order. For instance, the Shu points of the Large Intestine meridian are LI 1 (Shangyang), jing (well) point; LI 2 (Erjian), ying (spring) point; LI 3 (Sanjian), shu (stream) point; LI 5 (Yangxi), jing (river) point; and LI 11 (Quchi), the he (sea) point. These Shu points are the metal, water, wood, fire, and earth points respectively.

This twofold knowledge of how to predict the number of the jing (well), ying (spring), and shu (stream) points on a meridian, as well as how to assign elemental energies to them, is a useful skill that allows us to further understand the function of a point.

Also, understanding the elemental energy of the points fulfills several important functions. First, it provides an appreciation of the basic energy configuration of that point. For instance, HT 9 (Shaochong) is the wood point on a fire meridian. As such, it can be used to add or delete wood energy from the fire meridian. The nature of the wood element should come to mind here, that is, the point has a regenerative, spring-like quality to it. Second, the elemental energy of a point is not only related to the energy incarnated in that point but also to the meridian the point is on. To continue with the example of HT 9, the wood point on a fire meridian, the relationship between wood and fire is one of nourishment, promotion, and growth. It is what we would call the Tonification or Mother point of the meridian. Thus, HT 9 (Shaochong) can be used to tonify the Heart meridian. Tonification and Dispersion points are primary treatment sites on any meridian for building or reducing the energy in the organ-meridian complex. Needle technique accomplishes the tonification or dispersion.

An example of a dispersion point on the Heart meridian would be HT 7 (Shenmen), the shu (stream) point and the earth point. First, earth points assist in balancing; they can add or take away earth energy from the element in question and we can use the point in this way. Second, the relationship between earth and fire is one of the son who receives or takes energy from the mother. This is called the Dispersion or Sedation point. When this point is needled, it can balance the Heart and take excess energy from the Heart meridian.

Third, there is another interesting elemental relationship when the point in question has the same elemental energy as the meridian it is on. An example of this is HT 8 (Shaofu), the fire point on a fire meridian. The term for this type of point is the "horary point." Horary points always manifest the same elemental energy as the meridian they are on. In this case HT 8 (Shaofu) is a very "fiery" point. It can be used to add or take away fire from the meridian. *Table 12* below records the Tonification, Dispersion (Sedation), and Horary points of each meridian, and *Table 13* lists the points that corresponds to each element.

*Table 12.* Tonification, Dispersion, and Horary Points for the Twelve Main Meridians

| MERIDIAN | TONIFICATION | DISPERSION/SEDATION | HORARY |
|----------|--------------|---------------------|--------|
| Lung | LU 9 | LU 5 | LU 8 |
| Large Intestine | LI 11 | LI 2 | LI 1 |
| Stomach | ST 41 | ST 45 | ST 36 |
| Spleen | SP 2 | SP 5 | SP 3 |
| Heart | HT 9 | HT 7 | HT 8 |
| Small Intestine | SI 3 | SI 8 | SI 5 |
| Bladder | BL 67 | BL 65 | BL 66 |
| Kidney | KI 7 | KI 1 | KI 10 |
| Pericardium | PC 9 | PC 7 | PC 8 |
| Triple Warmer | TE 3 | TE 10 | TE 6 |
| Gall Bladder | GB 43 | GB 38 | GB 41 |
| Liver | LR 8 | LR 2 | LR 1 |

In addition to how points are classified, each point is significantly named and the point's use can be related to its name. A perusal of their translations shows that points are named in various ways. Some point names

*Table 13.* Elemental Energy of the Points

| MERIDIAN | WOOD | FIRE | EARTH | METAL | WATER |
|----------|------|------|-------|-------|-------|
| Lung | 11 | 10 | 9 | 8 | 5 |
| Large Intestine | 3 | 5 | 11 | 1 | 2 |
| Stomach | 43 | 41 | 36 | 45 | 44 |
| Spleen | 1 | 2 | 3 | 5 | 9 |
| Heart | 9 | 8 | 7 | 4 | 3 |
| Small Intestine | 3 | 5 | 8 | 1 | 2 |
| Bladder | 65 | 60 | 40 | 67 | 66 |
| Kidney | 1 | 2 | 3 | 7 | 10 |
| Pericardium | 9 | 8 | 7 | 5 | 3 |
| Triple Warmer | 3 | 6 | 10 | 1 | 2 |
| Gall Bladder | 41 | 38 | 34 | 44 | 43 |
| Liver | 1 | 2 | 3 | 4 | 8 |

carry an analogy to the earth, such as mountains and valleys. BL 60 (Kunlun), Kunlun Mountains, and LI 4 (Hegu), Meeting of the Valleys, are examples of this. Other points like LU 10 (Yuji), Fish Border, are analogous to animals. Architectural structures and astronomical and meteorological phenomena are represented in points such as CV 22 (Tiantu), Heaven Chimney, GV 23 (Shangxing), Upper Star, and GB 20 (Fengchi), Wind Pool. CV 12 (Zhongwan), Middle Stomach, ST 1 (Chengqi), Receives Tears, and CV 9 (Shuifen), Separates the Clear from the Turbid, indicate anatomical terms, therapeutic properties, and physiological/pathological changes. Yin/yang properties and theories of zang-fu and meridians are expressed in points such as GB 34 (Yanglingquan), Source of the Yang Mountain and SP 6 (Sanyinjiao), Crossroad of Three Yin.

Certainly there is no shortage of acupuncture books that provide various versions of the translated names of the points. Although all translations are subjective, they range from literal rigidity to loosely figurative interpretations. Some translations achieve a functional and insightful balance between the two extremes. The practitioner is encouraged to read books and consult other sources that can provide point names that will assist in understanding point function. The Appendix contains both a list of popular Chinese interpretations of the point names, which tends to emphasize the literal translation of the character,[4] and a French interpretation that strikes a good balance in conveying the spirit of the point.[5]

Case 2 provides a clinical example of one highly under-utilized, yet effective type of acupuncture point.

**Case 2.** Numbness treated through the jing (well) points

The patient's major complaint was one-sided numbness in the distal phalanxes of his thumb and index finger. This condition was accompanied by an electrical sensation that would occur when he lifted his arms over his head. The patient is a bronze worker who sits in a hunched position over his work which requires extremely fine and controlled hand movements. His hand was aggravated by overwork, stretching, and heavy work (such as yard work where his shoulders and arms were used excessively). He had received no Western medical diagnosis, although his condition resembled neurovascular compression of the brachial plexus.

The tongue was pale purple, flabby, scalloped, and slightly deviated to the left. The coat was wet, thick, yellow, and greasy. There were red dots on the tip, as well as cracks in the Lung area. The pulse was in the middle to superficial position, wiry, excessive, and fast. His Chinese diagnosis was qi and blood deficiency in the Lung and Large Intestine channels. The etiology was due to neurovascular compression or deficiency of the channels due to postural stress as well as an underlying Heart qi deficiency.

Points were needled along the course of the affected channels (Lung and Large Intestine), specifically LU 9 (Taiyuan), the influential point that dominates the vessels, and their jing (well) points, LU 11 (Shaoshang) and LI 1 (Shangyang) to activate the qi and blood. The Shixuan points of the thumb and index finger were also needled. In addition, a distal point, ST 12 (Quepen), was also treated with a needle to alleviate the neurovascular compression that was occurring because of occupationally induced poor posture.

After the first treatment, the numbness in the hand was immediately better. Feeling was restored to the thumb. Because of the patient's schedule, the next treatment was administered in two weeks. Following the second treatment, feeling was restored to both fingers.

Conscious postural improvement, the needle schema, and the application of Zheng Gu Shui along the course of the involved meridians to activate the flow of qi and blood completely resolved the numbness in five treatments. The patient was extremely satisfied with the results and was able to renew his work with no further or future impairment.

We should note that occupation and constitution may interfere with long-lasting results. The patient needs to be more conscious about his postural tension, which contributes to his major complaint. However, there are other constitutional weaknesses that were revealed during the interview that if strengthened, could enhance the effects of treatment. Such weaknesses include a history of heart disease and hypertension in the family. However, the patient preferred to end the course of treatment because of monetary considerations and the fact that he was satisfied with the treatment results.

4. Acupoints Research Committee of China, Society of Acupuncture and Moxibustion: *Brief Explanation of Acupoints of the 14 Regular Meridians*. Kai Z (trans). Beijing, PRC, 1987.

5. Darras JC: *Traite D'Acuponcture Medicale*, Tome I. Barnett M (trans). O.I.C.S. Newsletter, 1982; 1–35.

# CHAPTER 6

# LUO POINTS

## Special Vessels of Communication Between Channels

I f the body has an inherent wisdom—as centuries of Chinese clinical experience suggests—then surely the Luo points represent a facet of that wisdom. In classical Chinese acupuncture, Luo points are significant vehicles of treatment, although they seem to be less used in modern American acupuncture practice than one would expect given their historical, clinical usefulness. Part of the reason for this fact may be a predilection in American acupuncture colleges to deemphasize the classical energetics of points in favor of a more voluminous litany of point functions. Certainly, these functions are correct, but somehow they have become disassociated from their classical heritage. The intent of this chapter is to remind practitioners of the potency of one particular type of Antique point, the Luo points, and to demonstrate their value as a treatment option.

Classical literature reveals that there are three types of Luos referred to variously as lesser connecting or contributing channels or collaterals. They are the meridian (superficial), the blood, and the minute Luos. Each of these channels or vessels is responsible for establishing a network through which qi and blood can be sent to every part of the body.

Minute and blood Luos are very small vessels that arise from the main meridians but are too numerous and too small to be named or drawn as meridians.

They extend to every part of the body and infuse it with the qi and blood of life. *Figure 6* depicts a functional image of how these three Luos are interconnected and operate in the body.

The Luo points of the twelve main meridians can be used in two ways. Each way has a different therapeutic aim and each is manipulated by a different needle technique. Each Luo point activates a communication channel in two directions. One direction relates to the organ-meridian complex that the point is located on and is known as a longitudinal Luo. The second pathway connects the particular Luo point to the Source point of the coupled organ, and is known as a transverse Luo. In this way, the Luo points can be used to internally-externally balance the related organ-meridian complexes.

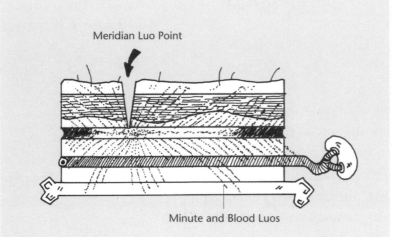

*Figure 6.* Meridian, Minute, and Blood Luos

The Luo points of the twelve main meridians connect the yin/yang pairs and assist in homeostatically regulating the yin/yang energy between the coupled channels. The Luo points do this at the periphery.

There are sixteen Luo points. Each of the twelve main meridians has a Luo point, which is located on the limbs. The Luo points of the Conception and Governing Vessels are located on the trunk. The Grand Luo of the Spleen is an additional Luo point and ST 18 (Rugen), opens to the great channel of the Stomach, another pathway between the Stomach and the Heart.

The additional Luo points of the Conception and Governing Vessels, and the Spleen and Stomach channels have other unique functions. At CV 15 (Jiuwei), the Luo point of the Conception Vessel Channel, the qi of all the yin channels converges, and likewise the qi of all of the yang channels concentrates at GV 1 (Changqiang), the Luo point of the Governing Vessel. All the blood of the body can be activated at SP 21 (Dabao), so this point is a handy tonic point particularly in the spring when the dormant energy of winter is regenerating and coming to the surface of the body. At ST 18 (Rugen) excess stomach energy may overflow into the upper chest.

The qi circulates through the superficial skin and muscle layers via the Luo channels before entering the primary channels. The connecting channels of the limbs travel toward their respective organs. Those of the Spleen and Stomach spread into the chest; the Ren (Conception Vessel) disperses into the abdomen; and the Du (Governing Vessel) separates into the head and the Bladder channel.

Luo channels are effective in treating chronic disorders of either the organ or the meridian. These disorders may be either excess or deficient in nature. The Chinese and the English methods are two primary ways of using Luo points for excess and deficient conditions. An analysis of these approaches reveals that the Luo points are used quite differently to either tonify or disperse the energy of the organ-meridian complex and yet clinically, each strategy works. A comparison and contrast of these methods is outlined below and summarized in *Table 14* for reference.

## Chinese Methods

According to the Chinese, the way to use the Luo points in cases of deficiency is with their coupled Source point. The rule is as follows: in cases of deficiency, tonify the Source point of the deficient meridian and disperse the Luo point of the coupled meridian. An application of this strategy applied to Lung deficiency would be to tonify LU 9 (Taiyuan), the Source point of

*Table 14.* Interpretations on Luo Point Use

| SOURCE | CONDITIONS | EXAMPLE AND NEEDLE TECHNIQUES | EXPLANATION | USE |
|---|---|---|---|---|
| **Chinese Methods** | **Deficiency** Tonify the Source point of the deficient meridian and disperse the Luo point of the coupled meridian | **Lung qi deficiency** Tonify LU 9 the Source point of the Lung meridian and disperse LI 6 the Luo point of its couple, the Large Intestine | Tonification of the Source point strengthens the "source" energy of a meridian. Dispersing the Luo point of the coupled channel opens the pathway between the Lung and the Large Intestine such that the husband-wife homeo-static relationship can be achieved | **Transverse Luo** Angle needle of the Luo point toward the Source point and disperse the Luo |
| | **Excess** For excess in a meridian disperse the Luo point of that meridian | **Lung excess** Disperse LU 7, the Luo point | Dispersing the Luo point of the affected meridian in cases of excess assists in draining excess energy from the meridian | **Longitudinal Luo** Angle needle along the course of the meridian in either direction with a dispersive technique |
| **English Methods** | **Deficiency** In deficiency, tonify the Luo point of the affected meridian and disperse the Source point of the coupled meridian | **Lung deficiency** Tonify the Luo point LU 7 and disperse the Source point of its coupled meridian LI 4 | Tonifying the Luo point is an effective treatment plan whereby to simulate the organ-meridian complex itself. Dispersing the Source points allows Source energy to be shared with the coupled meridian | **Transverse Luo** Angle needle of the Luo point with a dispersive technique toward the Source point to tonify |
| | **Excess** In case of fullness in the meridian, disperse the Source point | **Lung excess** Disperse the Source point LU 9 | A treatment strategy to remove excess energy | **Longitudinal Luo** Angle needle along the meridian, opposite the flow of energy, to disperse |

*As with any generalized treatment strategy, be sure that the signs and symptoms fit the clinical picture of the patient and make sense, instead of just subscribing to a formula.*

the Lung, the meridian affected by deficiency, and disperse LI 6 (Pianli), the Luo point of the Large Intestine, the coupled meridian of the Lung.

Most practitioners of Oriental medicine would agree that tonifying the Source point of a deficient meridian to supplement that deficiency makes sense. The added dimension of using Luo points may be new and not well understood, but the implication is that by using the Luo point to open the channel to the special vessel of communication between channels, homeostatic regulation can be attained between the husband and the wife. This means that the Lung can borrow energy from its yang partner of the same element. If the Large Intestine energy is sufficient or even excessive, it can be tapped to assist Lung function, thereby equilibrating the husband-wife relationship of the Lung and Large Intestine, two closely interconnected physiological systems. In this way, Luo points can be used as safety valves to send excess energy in one channel to replenish its deficient coupled channel. The needling strategy here is to use a tonification technique on LU 9 (Taiyuan) while dispersing LI 6 (Pianli).

However, in this case where the intent is not only to disperse but also to establish a connection between the Lung and Large Intestine, the Luo point is used transversely, that is, it is needled in the direction of the Source point. It is the needle placement that sets up the trajectory, the pathway between the Lung and the Large Intestine. See *Figure 7*, which illustrates the needle placement for transverse Luos.

In cases of excess in a particular organ-meridian complex, the aim of treatment with Luo points is to disperse the Luo point of the affected meridian. This approach should appear reasonable to practitioners who understand how to relieve excess. To treat excess in a meridian, disperse the Luo point of that meridian.

Again using the Lung meridian as the example, if the Lung is too full, disperse the Luo point of the Lungs, LU 7 (Lieque). Using the Luo point in this manner engages the longitudinal Luo, that is, we act on the organ-meridian complex itself, in order to drain it. In terms of needle

*T = Tonify*
*D = Disperse*
*⊥ = Perpendicular*

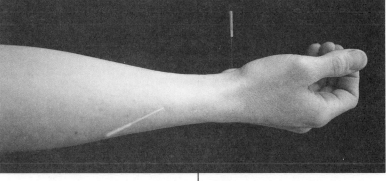

***Figure 7.*** Needle Placement for Transverse Luos in the Chinese Method

*T LU 9*
*D LI 6*

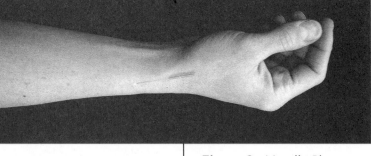

***Figure 8.*** Needle Placement for Longitudinal Luos in the Chinese Method

*D LU 7*

technique, a dispersion technique is applied to the point and the needle is angled along the course of the meridian in either direction. *Figure 8* depicts a needle placement for longitudinal Luos. Again, this is a therapeutic approach for dispersing the Luo that should make sense to most practitioners. What might be new, but should make sense, is the angle of the needle.

## English Sources

Acupuncture, which has its origins in classical Chinese medicine, assumed new nuances as it made its way to England via various countries, translations, and the soil and mind that assimilated it. Like the Chinese, the British use of the Luo points has guiding rules for tonifying deficiency and dispersing excess. A look at how they differ is quite useful.

According to the English acupuncture method, the rule is as follows: in deficiency, tonify the Luo point of the affected meridian and disperse the Source point of the coupled meridian. Continuing with the case of Lung deficiency, the Luo point of the Lung, LU 7 (Lieque), would be tonified and the Source point of its coupled meridian, LI 4 (Hegu), would be dispersed.

Analyzing this approach, we see that the meridians are still sharing their energy with each other; the difference lies in what is done to each point. In this system, the Luo channel of the deficient meridian is opened and strengthened, and creates a pathway whereby energy from its couple, which is being dispersed, can be brought to it. In this example, the Luo point is being used as a transverse vessel, that is, as a channel of communication between the Five Element pairs. To obtain the desired result, needle technique is critical: one point being tonified and another dispersed. In addition, the angle of insertion of the needle is also critical to open up the pathway between the two coupled meridians. *Figure 9* illustrates proper needle placement in the English method when Luos are used as transverse vessels.

In the case of excess in an affected meridian, the rule is, disperse the Source point.  Using the example of excess energy in the Lungs, LU 9 (Taiyuan), the Source point would be dispersed.  The mechanism for this strategy is depicted in *Figure 10*.

As I have mentioned, the Luo points of the twelve main meridians can be used to manipulate either longitudinal or transverse Luos.  Each has a different therapeutic aim and each is manipulated by a different needle technique.  The options are to use the Luo channels either longitudinally or transversely.  Luo points that are used as longitudinal vessels send a stimulus to their corresponding organ by way of the channel.  For instance, when LU 7 (Lieque), the Luo point of the Lungs, is stimulated longitudinally, the needle is inserted obliquely along the course of the Lung meridian in either direction.  Treating the point in this way stimulates the Lung organ-meridian complex and this is what is meant by using the point as a longitudinal Luo.  The sensation along the meridian should be very stimulating.

Luo points that are used as transverse channels have a horizontal trajectory that connects the Luo point of a meridian to the Source point of its coupled meridian.  In this way, Luo points internally-externally connect the coupled organ-meridian complexes so that the yin/yang organs are connected.  When we use the same Luo point

*T = Tonify*
*D = Disperse*
*⊥ = Perpendicular*

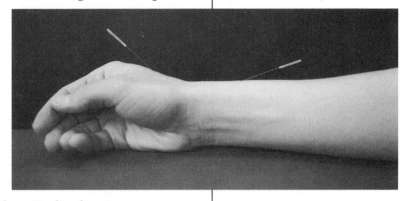

***Figure 9.*** Needle Placement for Transverse Luos in the English Method

*T LU 7*
*D LI 4 (angle of LI 4 needle could be ⊥.  Point here is to use a dispersion technique which could be achieved through other dispersion methods.)*

***Figure 10.*** Needle Placement for Longitudinal Luos in the English Method

*D LU 9*

of the Lung, LU 7 (Lieque), as a transverse channel, we communicate between the channels of the husband-wife couple through a special vessel. The Luo point allows us to tap into the Source point of the coupled meridian, the Large Intestine.

The Source point is sometimes referred to as the host, and the Luo point is termed the guest. Thus, the clinical utility of Luo points is either to stimulate the organ-meridian complex proper, or to connect to the source energy of the coupled meridian. The net effect of such a treatment strategy is an effective clinical approach that can be achieved easily without using too many needles.

We can sometimes observe the diagnostic patterns that the Luo points represent. We might notice signs of fullness such as rigidity or hardness, reddish colorations (heat), greenish or whitish colorations (cold retention). When the Luo points are deficient, signs such as flaccidity and indentations can also be noted.[1]

As well as giving the reasons for using the Luo points, Nguyen Van Nghi, M.D., points out that Luo vessels also have discrete channel symptoms that are similar to their organ pathologies. These symptoms are listed in *Table 15*.[2] Because they can stimulate the organs and various parts of the body and drain off excesses and supplement deficiency, Luo points should be part of every practitioner's repertoire.

*Case 3* offers a practical application of the use of a longitudinal Luo for excess conditions.

1. Maciocia G: *The Foundations of Chinese Medicine.* Churchill Livingston, London, 1989; p 152.

2. Van Nghi N: An exploration of the eight curious vessels. Lecture, Southwest Acupuncture College, Santa Fe, N.M., Sept., 1987.

*Table 15.* Nguyen Van Nghi on Luo Point Use

| MERIDIAN SYMPTOMATOLOGY | CONDITION | TREATMENT |
|---|---|---|
| hot palms (heat in hands), sneezing | LU fullness | disperse LU 7 (Luo) |
| enuresis | LU emptiness | tonify LU 9 (Source), disperse LI 6 (Luo) |
| pain in tooth | LI fullness | disperse LI 6 (Luo) |
| coldness in tooth | LI emptiness | tonify LI 4 (Source), disperse  LU 7 (Luo) |
| craziness, dementia, epilepsy | ST fullness | disperse ST 40 (Luo) |
| paralysis | ST emptiness | tonify ST 42 (Source), disperse SP 4 (Luo) |
| abdominal colic | SP fullness | disperse SP 4 (Luo) |
| swelling of abdomen | SP emptiness | tonify SP 3 (Source), disperse ST 40 (Luo) |
| thoracic pain | HT fullness | disperse HT 5 (Luo) |
| apnea, can't talk, immobility | HT emptiness | tonify HT 7 (Source), disperse SI 7 (Luo) |
| elbow mobility problems | SI fullness | disperse SI 7 (Luo) |
| eczema, furuncles, flaccid paralysis | SI emptiness | tonify SI 4 (Source), disperse HT 5 (Luo) |
| nasal obstruction, cephalgia, (headache that goes down face) | BL fullness | disperse BL 58 (Luo) |
| lumbago | BL emptiness | tonify BL 64 (Source), disperse KI 4 (Luo) |
| urinary retention, fecal retention | KI fullness | disperse KI 4 (Luo) |
| nosebleed, rhinnorhea | KI emptiness | tonify KI 3 (Source), disperse BL 58 (Luo) |
| cardialgia | PC fullness | disperse PC 6 (Luo) |
| stiffness in neck | PC emptiness | tonify PC 7 (Source), disperse TE 5 (Luo) |
| contraction of elbow | TE fullness | disperse TE 5 (Luo) |
| slackness of elbow articulation | TE emptiness | tonify TE 4 (Source), disperse PC 6 (Luo) |
| cold feet | GB fullness | disperse GB 37 (Luo) |
| laxity at the articulations of the foot | GB emptiness | tonify GB 40 (Source), disperse LR 5 (Luo) |
| lengthening of the penis and enlargement of the lips of the vagina | LR fullness | disperse LR 5 (Luo) |
| vaginal or scrotal puritis | LR emptiness | tonify LR 3 (Source), disperse GB 37 (Luo) |
| stiffness of spine | GV fullness | disperse GV 1 (Luo) |
| empty, light-headed, vertigo | GV emptiness | tonify GV 1 (Luo) |
| painful skin of abdomen | CV fullness | disperse CV 15 (Luo) |
| abdominal puritis, scratching | CV emptiness | tonify CV 15 (Luo) |
| general pain, a little bit everywhere, superficial on whole body | Grand Luo fullness | disperse SP 21 (Luo) |
| laxity of all the joints | Grand Luo emptiness | tonify SP 21 (Luo) |

*1. For deficiency of a meridian, tonify the Source point of the affected meridian and disperse the Luo point of the coupled meridian.  Example:  if Lung is insufficient, tonify LU 9 (Source point) and disperse LI 6 (Luo point), of the Coupled meridian.  When Large Intestine is deficient, tonify LI 4 (Source point) and disperse LU 7 (Luo point) of the Coupled meridian.*
*2. For fullness in a meridian, simply disperse the Luo of the meridian.*
*3. Meridians seek equilibrium automatically because of the Chinese clock dynamics, but the use of Luo points provides a shortcut to connecting interiorly/exteriorly related organ-meridians.*

**Case 3.**  Luo points in excess conditions

The patient was a forty-two-year-old medical doctor with a diagnosed case of multiple sclerosis. He had many problems that were part of his syndrome. His major complaint centered around extreme, erratic fatigue for the previous seven years. This fatigue was accompanied by several other problems that included the following: 1) leg spasticity and burning pain, 2) lack of bladder control with fluctuations between urgency and a weak stream and/or painful urinary retention, 3) blurry vision and spots before his eyes, 4) loss of balance, and 5) painful constipation and bowel cramps.

He had numerous other symptoms, but these were the characteristics of the complaint for which he had sought treatment. His tongue was red, thin, trembling, and slightly deviated. The sides and tip of the tongue were redder and rough. There were cracks in the stomach and chest areas. The tongue coat was thick, white, dry, and unrooted. Where there was no coating, the tongue had a glossy or mirror appearance.

His voice was quivery and weak; his lips were pale and sometimes slightly purple. He looked pale, tired, and usually felt hot on palpation. The pulse was slightly fast, deep, thin, and wiry with an irregular missed beat. The Lung, Kidney, and Liver positions were particularly deficient.

Because of the overall deficiency of his condition and the chronic nature of the complaint, I treated this patient for a period of two years, usually on a weekly basis. However, when acute, painful obstructions would develop due to underlying deficiencies, immediate results and relief were required. Under these circumstances, the patient was usually treated several times per week to remedy the condition. Several of these times when the patient complained of certain painful acute conditions, Luo points were selected as the points of choice because of their unique attributes.

In one classical usage, Luo points were used as channels to drain off or disperse excessive, stuck, or perverse energy.[3] Such excessive energy manifested as prostatitis, a sequela of his urinary disturbance. From time to time his prostate would become enlarged and produce symptoms of referred burning pain to the penis with perineal and suprapubic aching. In addition, he would experience urinary frequency, urgency, discomfort during urination, difficulty initiating the stream, nighttime urination, and an inability to ejaculate.

When this condition would develop, I tried several different approaches including Chinese herbs, Plum Blossom needling, and acupuncture, all of which worked. However, the two modalities that had both the most immediate as well as the most long lasting results included the use of two single points that I used alone or in combination depending upon his situation.

One point was the prostate/uterus point in the ear. On insertion of a needle into this point and a strong dispersion technique, the patient would report that he could immediately feel the burning, achiness, and referred pain diminish. This would occur in less than ten seconds. He would feel very relaxed, even sleepy, and enormously relieved from the pain. To hold the results, I would treat him three days in a row and that time frame appeared successful in setting in motion the reversal of his symptoms.

Another primary treatment point that worked very well was Liver 5 (Ligou), the Luo point of the Liver channel. To confirm the use of Liver 5 as the treatment point I would palpate the point as I do every point that I ever consider needling. Reaction at this point with a strong ah shi response indicated that the Liver channel was in excess. Remember that the Liver meridian encircles the external genitalia, hence this is one of the reasons why it was chosen over the Luo point of the Bladder or the Kidney. I needled this point in the direction of the meridian, using it as a longitudinal Luo to stimulate the channel, but with a strong dispersion technique to relieve the excess. Many times simply the strong palpation of the point brought about relief, but I always inserted a needle to strengthen the dispersion brought about by the palpation. In this way, the Luo point was one of the best points to use for draining the excess from the meridian.

3. Unschuld P: *Medicine in China, A History of Ideas.* University of California Press, Berkeley, 1985; pp 80–82.

# CHAPTER 7

# THE RULES OF POINT SELECTION AND GENERAL TREATMENT STRATEGIES

I n Chapter Five, I discussed how to select points based on the Chinese point classification system. In particular, that chapter outlined the potency of Command points. Through the analogy of different bodies of water I discussed the amount and type of qi each of these points contains. In addition, I discussed how to use these points seasonally both in a literal and figurative sense.

A discussion of how to select points for treatment is beneficial to beginning students of Chinese medicine, who usually lack the breadth and depth of clinical experience to support their choice of points. The outline that follows presents the parameters and the options for selecting points for treatment.

As students of Chinese medicine are well aware, it is customary in acupuncture colleges to receive copious clinical energetics compiled by practitioners from varied sources as well as from their own valuable clinical experience. However, without a sense of how points are classified and organized, students depend on memorizing or consulting notes instead of on a thinking process that is more in accord with the artistry of the diagnostic process and the patient's presentation. Neither of these can be found in any text. There are as many treatment options as there are patients and for that reason thinking and attentiveness must guide the practitioner to the correct treatment plan.

*Table 16* highlights a dozen different approaches that summarize the ways practitioners can think about how to select points for treatment. These methods are discussed below. Concomitantly, there are several different ways to execute needling strategy that student practitioners should keep in mind. Needle placement is never arbitrary: it is part of a treatment plan that should be executed in a logical and methodical order based on the aim of treatment as expressed in the treatment plan. These needling strategies are discussed following the rules of point selection.

*Table 16.* The Rules of Point Selection

| HOW TO SELECT POINTS FOR CLINICAL USE: |
| --- |
| Command points<br>   a. Seasonal disturbances (see Table 10)<br>   b. Classical Antique point usage (see Table 9) |
| Essential substance pathology (qi, blood, body fluid, jing, shen, and marrow deficiencies, stagnation, imbalances) |
| Unique energetics of each point |
| Name of the point |
| Pathway of the meridian |
| Chinese physiology and pathology (for instance, to treat Stomach ulcer, the Lung point in the ear is effective because the Lung controls mucous membranes) |
| Local and distal points |
| Five Seas (Nourishment, Blood, Qi (Energy), Marrow, and Internal Pollution) |
| Functional phases of points (active, passive, latent) |
| Organ-Meridian symptomatology |
| Organ interrelationships (therapeutic properties of the coupled channels in various diagnostic paradigms) |
| Understanding of Western science (anatomy, physiology, pathology) |

# Rules of Point Selection

1. Command points can be used for "seasonal" disturbances as well as for their classical antique point usage. An example of using a point seasonally would be to use LU 11 (Shaoshang). This point, the wood point on a metal meridian, can be needled for the "spring" of a condition, that is, one that has come on quickly. In this case, wood energy is excessive and is failing to control the blood, leading to symptoms of blood extravasation occurring in the metal meridian,

on which it is counteracting. Blood problems in the physiological domains that metal governs (i.e., nose, throat, chest) develop with pathological conditions such as epistaxis and hemoptysis.

2. Points can be selected that treat the pathologies of essential substances (qi, blood, body fluid, jing, shen, and marrow) with their deficiencies, stagnations, rebelliousness, or sinkingness—for example, CV 6 (Qihai) for KI qi xu (qi deficiency).

3. Points have peculiar, special energetics that distinguish them from other points; for example, GV 20 (Baihui) raises sinking Spleen qi.

4. The names of the points suggest ways in which to use them. For example, SP 6 (Sanyinjiao) is the meeting of the Three Leg Yin meridians and those meridians can be effectively treated through this point. See Appendix, "Translations of the Point Names," for a comprehensive list of all of the names of the points according to two sources.

5. The pathway of the meridian that has both internal and external manifestations can be used as the basis for point consideration. For example, CV 12 (Zhongwan) is a possible point for treatment of vertical headache because the Liver meridian ends at CV 12 (Zhongwan) and Liver headaches typically manifest at the top of the head.

6. An understanding of Chinese physiology and pathology provides unique insights into the functioning of the human body and how to treat it with certain points. For example, to treat a stomach ulcer the Lung point in the ear is extremely effective because according to zang-fu theory, the Lung controls the mucous membranes and stomach ulcer is a problem in the wearing down of the inner mucosa of the stomach.

7. For excess conditions, a combination of local and distal points is an effective treatment strategy. For example, select Command points that are major distal points for an area of dysfunction. Select local points

such as Mu or Shu points that are close to an organ and the sphere of energy that it controls. In the case of migraine, for instance, GB 41 (Zulinqi), a distal point, with GB 20 (Fengchi), a local point, is a good combination.

8. Activate the Five Seas, which pertain to energetic zones of the body. The Five Seas and the level of the body they are involved with are listed below.

*The Sea of Nourishment* assists in food absorption. It can be activated when the person has overeaten or is hungry or undernourished. Its points are ST 30 (Qichong) and ST 36 (Zusanli).

*The Sea of Blood* can tonify deficient blood or move blood stagnation. The Sea of Blood points are ST 37 (Shangjuxu), BL 11 (Dazhu), SP 10 (Xuehai), BL 17 (Geshu), and ST 39 (Xiajuxu).

*The Sea of Energy,* also referred to as the *Sea of Qi,* is activated by immediately usable points, reservoirs of energy that can be tapped. They are CV 6 (Qihai), ST 9 (Renying), CV 17 (Tanzhong), BL 10 (Tianzhu), and GV 14 (Dazhui).

*The Sea of Marrow* assists in strengthening the brain and the mind. Its points include GB 39 (Xuanzhong), GV 15 (Yamen), 16 (Fengfu), and 20 (Baihui).

*The Sea of Internal Pollution* refers to organs that help the body rid itself of waste. They are the Lung, Kidney, Bladder, and Large Intestine organs. Use their respective points.

9. Points possess various functional phases that are manifestations of their health. Active points are those that are active or that spontaneously fire because of their pathology. They represent a problem in the physiology of a particular point. For example, a pre-appendicitis condition may be detected by a throbbing sensation at Lanwei, the appendix reflex point. Likewise, sinus congestion may be signified by pressure in the BL 2 (Zanzhu), ST 1 (Chengqi), and ST 2 (Sibai) areas.

Passive points are those points that only react when they are mechanically stimulated or aroused through pressure. For example, a patient with Spleen qi xu and damp generally has exquisite tenderness at SP 4 (Gongsun) whether the manifestations of Spleen qi xu with damp are overt or preclinical.

Latent points are those that are neither active nor passive. They indicate that the function of each point is healthy and not a problem. The more latent points there are, the healthier the person is. These points can be selected not so much to correct pathology as to enhance bodily function.

10. Specific organ-meridian symptomatology is clearly associated with each organ-meridian complex that suggests point use. For instance, the Large Intestine organ-meridian complex clearly deals with intestinal problems. Likewise, because the channel traverses the shoulder area, LI 15 (Jianyu) can be used for shoulder problems and LI 4 (Hegu) is indicated for tooth problems because its meridian traverses the mouth area.

11. The therapeutic properties of a point may be modified by the organ-meridian complex it is coupled with. For example,
   a.  the Lung meridian may be treated alone, or
   b.  in combination with the Large Intestine because of its Five Element relationship, or
   c.  combined with the Spleen meridian by virtue of its Six Division association, or
   d.  used with the Kidney meridian because of extraordinary meridian and zang-fu energetics.

12. An understanding of Western anatomy, physiology, pathology, and other clinical sciences can shed light on point selection. For example, ST 36 (Zusanli) can be chosen to adjust indigestion from excess or deficient hydrochloric acid secretion.

## Selection of Treatment Strategies

This list of possibilities does not imply that only one paradigm can be chosen when a treatment plan of points is being generated.  Rather, it simply gives some guidelines to assist the practitioner in choosing points.  The process of initiating treatment, as I have said, is a highly logical procedure within the Chinese healthcare delivery system.  Point selection follows the treatment plan, which follows diagnosis.  But diagnosis is a highly sophisticated art involving the synthesis of all of the data gained by asking questions, palpating the pulse and the body, auscultation, olfaction, inspection, and numerous other parameters.  This integration, while logical, is both artful and intuitive in the sense that intuition is knowledge based upon the integration of perceptions.

Beginning students of Oriental medicine can be overwhelmed by all the methods that can be used to establish the basis for a diagnosis, never mind the complexity of weaving that information into a whole that addresses the person's problem.  Students assiduously strive to cover everything that must be mastered in order to know as much as possible about the person, and this is learned well in schools.  What takes longer, and what is generally only grasped in clinical practice, is where to begin with treatment of the person—how to grasp the essence of the person, the root of the problem, and the way in which to initiate the treatment process.  This ability may be a function of experience and alacrity on the part of the observant practitioner who attunes the individual presence of the patient to her or his own individual skill as a physician.  However, a few general treatment principles can be advanced for the beginning practitioner of Oriental medicine and these can assist the practitioner and the patient in their discovery of balance.

The first and golden rule of treatment should always

be to do no harm. This maxim demands much skill, honesty, precision, and humbleness on the part of practitioners to treat what they are comfortable in treating. There must also be an awareness of the seriousness of illness; their own scope of knowledge and practice; and an understanding of the intricacies of organ interrelationships, needle technique, point location, herbal, dietary, and other lifestyle considerations. There must be an integrity of spirit and a willingness to learn and develop skills to meet ever-changing medical problems and the complexity and uniqueness of each individual patient. There must be total attentiveness and mindfulness during every step of the intake and the delivery system and a knowledge of when to refer if the case exceeds the practitioner's ability. If the practitioner treats to the best of her ability with this guideline "to do no harm" in mind, she will encompass the spirit of a physician. Many times "doing no harm" for the average practitioner means not doing too much in a treatment. Yet doing no harm implies doing what the practitioner should be able to accomplish; the other part of this maxim is its correlate—to do the best we can.

With these guidelines as the automatic operating assumptions on the part of the patient and the practitioner, practitioners then need to formulate an overall strategy with which to accomplish their objectives. Point selection and needling strategies must be adopted if acupuncture is part of the therapeutic modality. Practitioners have numerous historical positions from which to adopt a treatment strategy. *Table 17* summarizes the needle strategies that can be considered after point selection has occurred.

| *Table 17.* Needling Strategies |
|---|
| Treat both the major complaint and the accompanying symptoms within the context of the whole person. |
|    a) Know when to treat the acute condition, when to treat the chronic, when the acute is a manifestation of the chronic; that is: when to treat the root, or treat the branch, or treat the root and the branch. |
|    b) Know when to disperse a pathogenic factor, when to reduce. |
|    c) Know when to strengthen the body, when to reinforce. |
|    d) Differentiate the problem with the diagnostic framework of choice. |
| Be efficient with point selection. |
| Choose clinically effective points. |
| Generally insert needles from top to bottom to bring the energy down. In emergency conditions, however, sometimes the energy needs to be raised, and then the needles are inserted from bottom to top. |
| Insert needles from front to back, from right to left, from the midline to the lateral aspect, and remove in the order that they were inserted. |
| Insert needles singularly for their known abilities. |
| Insert needles in a chain of points. |
| Encircle a point with needles. |
| Needle the points on the upper extremities first, then on the lower, and from exterior to interior to bring the yang to the interior (yin). This action will tonify. |

# Needling Strategies

1. Three major orientations cover all the diseases that will be clinically encountered. They are treating the root, treating the branch (manifestation), and treating both the root and the branch.

Treating the root is perhaps the purest of all treatment strategies. It embodies the Chinese emphasis on ameliorating the underlying problem in order to restore the patient to balance. This approach can be used especially if the clinical signs and symptoms are not severe. There are numerous treatment styles within this approach and all aim at correcting the root imbalance. These styles include balancing the pulses, eliminating navel tension, or reducing the number of passive and active points in the body. Although the scope of this book is not to outline how the root is perceived or corrected in the individual, it is important to note that failure to treat the root in many cases represents a symptomatic approach to medicine and may provide only minimal relief.

Treating the branch (that is, the manifestations) has its place in the scheme of treatment. This is a beneficial and indeed appropriate treatment strategy when the problem is acute and/or life threatening in nature. The patient's problem demands that it be dealt with immediately. This approach necessitates a spirit of compassion and an ability to perceive the causes of signs and symptoms. It is Chinese emergency medicine at its best.

"Treat the root and treat the branch (manifestation)," is an effective treatment plan that is used most often by most practitioners. This approach simultaneously acknowledges both the presenting complaint of the person as well as the root cause of the disorder. It is used for chronic conditions and constitutes an efficient treatment strategy as long as the practitioner has the ability to see how the manifestations of the symptoms are connected to the root of the problem.

Regardless of which approach is selected, all treatment styles require that both the major complaint and the accompanying symptoms be addressed within the context of the whole person. The practitioner must learn to discern when to treat the acute condition, when to treat the chronic condition, and when the acute is a manifestation of the underlying, chronic problem. As in good herbal medicine, points are chosen for how they work together to treat the pattern of the illness. Neither points nor herbs should be used to treat each sign and symptom without considering the whole pattern.

2. Other treatment approaches are important to bear in mind as well. Skilled practitioners who do no harm and also do the best they can must have the wisdom to know when to disperse a pathogenic factor and when to strengthen the body, that is, when to reinforce, when to reduce, and when not to be redundant. They must be able to discern whether the problem is one of the zang-fu, the essential substances, the

jing luo, and so on. Once a proper differentiation is made based on the theoretical framework that the practitioner adopts, a treatment plan must be formulated that matches the chosen diagnostic framework and the related, selected points. Needle technique must match intent.

For beginning students of acupuncture, this step often feels overwhelming. It can be difficult to know what is going on with the patient when so much information needs to be assimilated. Two major pitfalls that students can succumb to are what can be called the shotgun approach on the one hand, and tunnel vision on the other.

With the shotgun approach, instead of a precise, discerning diagnosis, there is a tendency to think that everything is involved. Because it is difficult for beginning practitioners to see the bigger picture of patterns and interrelationships, their treatment strategies tend to be imprecise and unfocused. They try to do too much, so the range of their treatments is too wide to be effective. By trying to treat every symptom beginners end up treating very little.

Tunnel vision is the opposite of the shotgun approach. There is again the fundamental problem of not seeing the larger picture—the patterns and interrelationships. However, instead of trying to do too much, the practitioner focuses myopically on one thing. For example, the practitioner may always assume that knee problems mean Kidney problems and therefore hone in on only one facet of the case.

The balance between these two extremes is the ability to see the pattern of the pathogenesis. Points are chosen for their synergistic effects, that is, for how they work together to treat the pattern of the illness, not just the symptoms.

3. Point selection must be efficient. Choose points with a multiplicity of functions that will meet the therapeutic aim. Clinical experience seems to bear out

that "less is more and more is less," meaning an economy of points often achieves more than choosing too many points. The practitioner must try to see the common denominator, the congruence between points that are selected and the essence of the person.

Points should be selected that meet the diagnostic criteria. My preference is to use few points and to use only those that are directly related to the treatment plan. Because few points are chosen so as not to con-fuse the redirecting of the body's energy, points with a multiplicity of energetics are the most efficient. Again, we choose points for their synergistic effects, that is, for how they work together to treat the whole pattern of illness.

4. Clinically effective points may be chosen—that is, points with known therapeutic value. Clinically effec-tive points may be points on the fourteen meridians or points that are part of the Extra point system.

5. In most cases of tonification, needles should be inserted from top to bottom to bring the energy down, to root and secure it. For example, when there is too much energy in the head or upper part of the body, points should be selected from the lower part of the body. Infantile convulsion and migraine are effectively treated this way with points such as KI 1 (Yongquan) and GB 41 (Zulinqi) respectively. However, there are instances in emergency situations—such as fainting—when the clear qi does not rise and the treatment points such as GV 26 (Shuigou) on the top of the body and HT 9 (Shaochong) on the extremities are indicated.

6. Other treatment directives include first treating the front and then the back; treating the right before the left; and needling from the midline to the lateral side. The theoretical justification for this is to bring yin (front/right/middle) into yang (back/left/lateral). (For example, if CV 12 [Zhongwan] and ST 21 [Liangmen] are being needled, needle CV 12 first and then ST 21.) Then, withdraw the needles in the order of insertion.

7.  Needle the points on the upper extremities first and then on the lower, and/or needle from the exterior to the interior and then remove the needles in the order they were inserted, as above.  The justification for this is to bring yang into yin.

8.  Needle each point singularly for its unique energetics, for example, SP 6 (Sanyinjiao) for edema of the lower limbs.

9.  Needle a chain of points along a meridian or in an affected area to strengthen the therapeutic aim.  For example, for Gall Bladder sciatica, needle GB 30 (Huantiao), 34 (Yanglingquan), 40 (Qiuxu), and 44 (Zuqiaoyin).

10.  Encircle a point with needles.  For example, the navel, which should not be needled directly, can be treated by needling all around the area (see *Figure 11*).

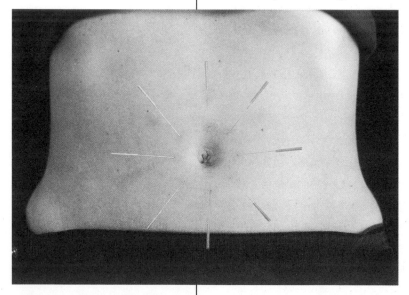

*Figure 11.* Needling Around a Point

*Case 4* offers an example of using a particular treatment strategy to achieve improvement.

**Case 4.** The use of distal points for knee pain

The patient was a forty-five-year-old woman whose major complaint was traumatic arthritis on the medial side of her knee, exacerbated by her occupation as a gardener. She did much of her work on her knees without protection. In addition, she had tendonitis of the arms, calcification of the elbow, and low back pain. Apart from her major complaint, the patient presented with a condition of agitation and stress. Because of money concerns, she wanted quick results. She was highly resistant to answering any questions that she felt were not relevant to the major complaint and also insisted that needles be inserted at her knee.

My approach was to ask many of the traditional questions and to do a thorough physical exam to assess the root of the problem. The patient's demand for quick resolution of the problem challenged my ability to determine the root cause of the disease. Finally, because of her uncooperative attitude about the questioning and about the tongue and pulse examinations, I selected palpation of the abdomen and the knee to ascertain etiology. The patient still could not understand why attention was being placed on the abdomen, but I was adamant about this particular procedure.

Needles were placed locally around the knee in the first treatment. However, the emotionally volatile patient clearly reported that she could feel more benefit from the distal points used to rectify abdominal tension, discomfort, or deficiency. After the first treatment, the patient was considerably less demanding and demonstrative and told me to do whatever I thought was necessary. The knee, back, and tendonitis all felt better, and by the fourth treatment the patient effusively thanked me for her relief and vowed she would be back at the slightest sign of aggravation.

Three years later the patient returned to the college clinic for manifestations of stress. The original major complaint that brought her to me was a thing of the past. This is an example of a treatment strategy in which the local area was not the area of choice for treatment. More distal points that affect that area for other reasons corrected the root in less than four treatments.

# The Treatment of Headaches with Unusual Clinically Effective Points, Local and Distal Points

Millions of people endure headaches on a daily basis. While some cope relatively successfully, mainly with analgesics, for others this pain is an inescapable fact of life. Books on the treatment of disease more than adequately recognize this affliction that characterizes the human condition and suggest various treatment strategies for the different types of headaches that can occur and they can be consulted. However, there are other useful treatment approaches not found in the classical literature that are based on additional differentiations discussed below. *Table 18* lists six common types of headache, their corresponding zang-fu differentiation, and their primary treatment points not found in classical literature.

**Table 18.** The Treatment of Headaches with Unusual Points Not Found in Classical Literature

| TYPE OF HEADACHE | ZANG-FU DIFFERENTIATION | POINT USE |
|---|---|---|
| Vertical | Liver | CV 12 (Zhongwan) |
| Band type | Spleen qi xu with damp | CV 12 (Zhongwan) |
| Frontal | Yangming (ST/LI) | CV 12 (Zhongwan) |
| Behind ears | Triple Warmer | CV 12 (Zhongwan) |
| Occipital | Bladder | BL 40 (Weizhong) |
| Temporal | Gall Bladder/Triple Warmer | TE 9 (Sidu) and GB 36 (Waiqiu) |

*Explanations:*

*The Liver and Spleen meridians intersect at CV 12. The Large Intestine and Triple Warmer meridians also pass through CV 12. The Stomach meridian begins at CV 12.*

*BL 40 pulls energy out of the head.*

*TE 9 and GB 36 are Xi (cleft) points, points of accumulation or blockage.*

The rationale for using each point is given in *Table 18* and is well justified, but obviously these are rather uncommon points. The treatment of headache with these unusual points illustrates how important it is to understand the internal pathways of meridians, an understanding that opens up new and clearly effective treatment strategies. As I have discussed in other sections in this book, the major treatment point may be used either alone or as the primary point in a broader treatment plan.

Before using these points, we must decide how to needle them. For instance, for a headache at the vertex, CV 12 (Zhongwan) is the recommended point. However, should the point be tonified or dispersed? The answer, of course, depends on the nature of the headache at the vertex. For instance, if the headache has strong pounding pain, it is due to Liver yang rising, so CV 12 would be dispersed. If there is emptiness or even cold, the headache is from blood deficiency, so CV 12 would be tonified.

The same would hold true for differentiating a frontal headache. If the headache is dull and nagging, it could be from qi deficiency, so CV 12 would be tonified. If there is stuffiness or nausea, the headache could be from food stagnation, so the point would be dispersed.  By understanding the different types of pain and the functional spheres of the zang-fu organs, the practitioner can formulate a diagnosis, the treatment plan, and the appropriate needle technique.

**Case 5.** Food poisoning headache treated with a combination of local and distal points

The patient had just arrived at my clinic for a weekly treatment and was experiencing an acute stomach-ache.  She had lunch at a small fast-food restaurant with questionable sanitary conditions.  She was doubled over in pain, which was spasmodic and colicky.  She also had an intense, pounding frontal headache that was making her nauseous.

With the patient in a reclining position, I applied a strong dispersion technique to ST 34 (Liangqiu), the Xi (cleft) point of the Stomach meridian.  Within a few minutes the stomach pain stopped.  However, she still had the headache, so I continued to work on CV 12 (Zhongwan), the influential point that dominates all the fu organs as well as being the Front Mu point of the Stomach.  Shortly thereafter, the headache and nausea also stopped and the patient was able to leave the office feeling fine.

# CHAPTER 8

# SIX DIVISION TREATMENTS

In the treatment of acute conditions, whether internal or musculoskeletal, practitioners strive to choose points whose therapeutic effectiveness has been established. Such options may fall into any category of points in the point classification system. One group of points that possesses unique functions for acute conditions are the Xi (cleft) points.

Xi (cleft) points are points of accumulation or blockage. They are considered reflex points of the organ-meridian complex; that is, their tenderness indicates problems in that complex. They exhibit spontaneous or passive characteristics when there is a blockage or accumulation in the corresponding organ-meridian complex.

An interesting approach to these conditions is the use of the "Six Divisions" as energetic layers to treat these problems. In this system, the use of the Xi (cleft) points of the meridians paired together in Six Division diagnosis are the points employed. This treatment strategy reflects the Chinese cosmological view of "as above, so below." This expression means that both the organ-meridian complex impaired above (upper part of the body) and the corresponding complex below (lower part of the body) will tend to be affected in acute conditions because of their Six Division coupling. This treatment strategy illustrates both how to use the organ-meridian complexes paired in the Six Divisions with the traditional use of Xi (cleft) points as points of accumulation or blockage. *Table 19* lists the Six Divisions and their associated Xi (cleft) points.

*Table 19.* The Six Divisions, Associated Xi (cleft) Points, and the Side of the Body to Needle

| DIVISION | XI (CLEFT) POINTS | SIDE OF BODY |
|---|---|---|
| Taiyang (SI/BL) | SI 6 (Yanglao)<br>BL 63 (Jinmen) | Left<br>Left |
| Shaoyang (TE/GB) | TE 7 (Huizong)<br>GB 36 (Waiqiu) | Right<br>Left |
| Yangming (ST/LI) | LI 7 (Wenliu)<br>ST 34 (Liangqiu) | Right<br>Right |
| Taiyin (LU/SP) | LU 6 (Kongzui)<br>SP 8 (Diji) | Right<br>Right |
| Jueyin (LR/PC) | LR 6 (Zhongdu)<br>PC 4 (Ximen) | Left<br>Left |
| Shaoyin (KI/HT) | HT 6 (Yinxi)<br>KI 5 (Shuiquan) | Left<br>Right and/or Left |

A specific clinical example of an internal problem in which this strategy could be used would be a patient who presents with an acute case of daytime asthma. There is shortness of breath with more difficulty on the exhale, wheezing due to phlegm, cough, tenderness at LU 1 (Zhongfu), and a slippery Lung pulse. It is apparent that the Lung is the affected organ. In this case, the Xi (cleft) point of the Lung, Lung 6 (Kongzui), combined with the Xi (cleft) point of the Spleen, SP 8 (Diji) is chosen.

Needle technique involves applying a dispersion technique to both Xi (cleft) points. Lung 6 and Spleen 8 are needled on the right-hand side because the energetics of the Lung and Spleen are primarily right sided (see my discussion of commonly accepted pulse assignments in Chapter Fourteen). The reason a dispersion technique is employed is to break up the accumulation or blockage in the lungs as indicated by the phlegm. Needling is performed unilaterally and in this example is all on the right side, although this would not be the case for all of the Xi (cleft) points, which can be seen when the pulse assignment chart is consulted. For added convenience, the side of the body to needle is also listed in *Table 19*.

Needle technique is matched with the treatment strategy, that is, we should apply strong dispersion techniques to the accumulation points. Needles need not be retained. An in-and-out technique with appropriate dispersion is all that is required. These points may either be used alone or as the skeletal basis of a treatment that addresses the major complaint.

Another example that involves the Lung/Spleen pair would be a case of acute dysmenorrhea, where the etiology of the painful period is stagnation due to blood deficiency. Spleen 8, the Xi (cleft) point, is chosen because of the accumulation or blockage that the painful period represents. In this case, the Spleen is failing to control the blood. Not enough blood is being produced and in turn this deficit is leading to stagnation. According to the Six Division model of "as above, so below," Lung 6, the paired Xi (cleft) point, is also selected.

*Table 20* presents common acute clinical conditions and the appropriate Six Division Xi (cleft) points that would be used for those cases. Some commonly used supplementary points, to be added according to signs and symptoms, are also included.

The Six Division framework is probably better known for use in other contexts. The *Shang Han Lun (Treatise of Cold-Induced Disorders)* outlines the progression of symptoms of a cold pathogen that has invaded the body and how those signs and symptoms change as the pathogen makes its way through these various energetic layers.[1] French acupuncturist Yves Requena uses the Six Division paradigm to extrapolate on various personality/constitutional types that correspond to these energetic zones.[2] More information on these

---

1. Hsu H-Y: *Shang Han Lun.* Oriental Healing Arts Institute, Los Angeles, 1981.

2. Requena Y: *Terrains and Pathology,* Vol. 1. Paradigm Publications, Brookline, Mass., 1986.

approaches can be found by consulting the reference material cited in the footnotes. The system described in this chapter represents another classical Chinese use of the Six Division model, an elegant, understated treatment strategy that yields dramatic and effective results when appropriately selected.

*Table 20.* Common Acute Clinical Conditions, their Corresponding Six Division Level, Xi (cleft) Points, and Supplementary Points

| CONDITION | SIX DIVISION LEVEL AND XI (CLEFT) POINTS | SUPPLEMENTARY POINTS |
|---|---|---|
| Acute Liver problems, menstrual problems | Jueyin: PC 4, LR 6 | LR 5 (Ligou) |
| Acute lumbago, declining eyesight in the elderly | Taiyang: SI 6, BL 63 | BL 1 (Jingming) |
| Acute menstrual problems (dysmenorrhea) or those due to qi and blood stagnation | Taiyin: LU 6, SP 8 | SP 10 (Xuehai) |
| Any blockage | Shaoyang: TE 7, GB 36 | PC 6 (Neiguan) |
| Bleeding anywhere | Taiyin: LU 6, SP 8 | — |
| Chest pain, obesity, and heart disease | Jueyin: PC 4, LR 6 | KI 9 (Zhubin) |
| Hysteria, angina | Shaoyin: HT 6, KI 5 | KI 9 (Zhubin) |
| Infantile convulsion | Taiyang: SI 6, Bl 63 | KI 1 (Yongquan) |
| Mastitis | Yangming: LI 7, ST 34 | Ear: Liver, Endocrine, Mammary glands, Shenmen |
| Prostatitis | Shaoyin: HT 6, KI 5 | CV 3 (Zhongji), BL 62 (Shenmai) |
| Rage | Shaoyang: TE 7, GB 36 | — |
| Uterine hemorrhage (life threatening) | Taiyin: LU 6, SP 8 | SP 1 (Yinbai) LR 1 (Dadun) |

*Case 6* illustrates the use of the Six Division framework for a common clinical condition, backache.

**Case 6.** Six Divisions: an energetic, philosophical model for pain and blockage

The patient was a thirty-nine-year-old male who was experiencing an acute case of lumbago from trauma to the back. This condition was brought about by vigorous exercise. He had not worked out strenuously in a long time and had a history of minor episodes of back strain usually brought on by lifting heavy objects, a common cause of acute lumbago.

For this patient, the usual treatment after such an injury would be rest, hot baths with relaxing bath salts, the application of Chinese liniments and bruise plasters, all of which would give some relief for a certain time. On this particular occasion, the back strain was quite severe and six weeks later he still had not recovered. He sought the assistance of an acupuncturist.

In this particular case, I opted to choose a more distal point mostly because I was treating the person out of the office, but also because of the effectiveness of the points selected. The Six Division framework was selected, and I chose SI 6 (Yanglao) and BL 63 (Jinmen), the Xi (cleft) points that specifically treat acute lumbago.

SI 6 (Yanglao), in the upper part of the body, was needled first on the left side. The point was needled with a thick needle and a strong stimulus—that is, a dispersive technique—in the direction of the flow of the meridian. The patient felt strong energy go up his arm. At the same time the patient was instructed to mobilize his back by standing and swaying to activate the affected area. His back immediately felt better even though he had endured six weeks of pain that ranged from immobilizing to residual discomfort.

To consolidate the effect, BL 63 (Jinmen), the corresponding Xi (cleft) point, was also needled on the left side against the flow of energy in the meridian. However, the effect was not as strong as with SI 6 because SI 6 had acted so well. The needles were retained only for the time it took to achieve the desired needle sensation and to note the improvement. After this treatment the patient said that his back was fine.

# EIGHT NEEDLE TECHNIQUE

**B**ack pain is part of the human condition. From any therapeutic perspective, this problem can be understood as the result of the trauma and stress to which the back is normally subject, and the treatment of low back pain is one of the chief complaints for which practitioners are consulted. This complex condition can be difficult to resolve because of its numerous causes, but if the diagnosis is correct, successful treatment is possible. From a Chinese perspective, back pain has a close but not exclusive functional relationship to the Kidney, the source of life, and hence such a disorder can serve as a reflection of the vitality of the Kidney, the Gate of Life.

In the case of low back pain from deficiency of Kidney qi and yang, the "Eight Needle Technique" is particularly effective. The doctors I studied with in China maintained that Chinese needles must be employed in this treatment strategy to most effectively nourish the Kidney energy and circulate the qi and blood (because this is their only experience). However, it has been my and my students' experience on hundreds of patients that Japanese needles, even #1 Seirins, can achieve therapeutic results. *Table 21* lists the points used in Eight Needle Technique, their corresponding angles, and depths of needle insertion. Following the table, the primary energetics that contribute to making this formula effective in the treatment of low back pain due to Kidney qi and yang deficiency are discussed.

Note that many of the energetics delineated here pertain to symptoms of Kidney qi and yang xu and as such are not limited to the manifestation of low back pain. Consequently, by treating Kidney qi and yang xu through these points, there are many added benefits in addition to alleviating back pain. This formula can also be modified if back pain is not the major complaint (for example, by eliminating BL 40) so as to strengthen the qi of the Kidney. This treatment in turn will benefit many of the domains belonging to Kidney function in Oriental medicine.

*Table 21.* Eight Needle Technique: Points, Locations, Angles, and Depths of Insertion

| POINTS | LOCATIONS | ANGLES AND DEPTHS OF INSERTION |
|---|---|---|
| BL 23 Shenshu (bilateral) | 1.5 cun lateral to the lower border of the spinous process of the 2nd lumbar vertebra | Perpendicular .8 in.–1 in. |
| GV 4 Mingmen | In the depression below the lower border of the spinous process of the 2nd lumbar vertebra | Perpendicular .5 in.–1 in. Moxa needle or the moxa box may also be applied here |
| BL 25 Dachangshu (bilateral) | 1.5 cun lateral to the lower border of the spinous process of the 4th lumbar vertebra | Perpendicular .8 in.–1.5 in. |
| GV 3 Yaoyanguan | In the depression below the spinous process of the 4th lumbar vertebra level with the iliac crest | Perpendicular .5 in.–1 in. |
| BL 40 Weizhong (bilateral) | At the popliteal crease of the knee between the tendons of the muscles biceps femoris and semitendinosus | Perpendicular .5 in.–1.5 in. or bleed No moxa |

# Clinical Energetics of the Eight Needle Technique Points

As the Back Shu point of Kidney, BL 23 (Shenshu) tonifies and regulates the qi of the Kidney. It is good for strengthening the Kidney's reception of qi in cases of chronic asthma and benefits the ears in tinnitus or deafness.  It is good for chronic eye disorders such as blurred vision, prolapse of the kidney, weak legs, and irregular menses.  It resolves dampness in the lower burner and strengthens the lower back.

Bladder 23 (Shenshu) is better for tonifying the yang aspect of Kidney qi, but it can also be used for Kidney yin deficiency.  Consequently, it can be used for yang pathologies such as lack of sexual desire, lack of will power, negativity, lack of initiative, depression, dizziness, poor memory, blurred vision, fatigue, constant desire to sleep, cold knees, renal colic, and nephritis.  Yin deficiencies that it can treat include tidal fever, seizures, and infantile paralysis.

BL 23 (Shenshu) nourishes Kidney essence making the point useful in impotence, nocturnal emissions, infertility, and spermatorrhea.  It benefits the bones and marrow and is good for any bone pathology.  Because it nourishes the blood, it can be used for anemia, brightening the eyes, and alopecia.

The Gate of Life, GV 4 (Mingmen), encompasses Kidney yin and yang, which are inextricably bound together.  Therefore, GV 4 is appropriate for the two aspects of Kidney qi deficiency, that is, Kidney yin and yang.  Mingmen tonifies the original qi of the Kidney.  In this capacity it nourishes the original qi of preheaven, that is, the person's constitution, basic vitality, and genetic inheritance on a physical and mental level.

Mingmen is the most powerful point to strengthen Kidney yang and all the yang in general, especially if combined with moxa.  It tonifies and warms the "Fire of the Gate of Vitality," resolving Kidney yang xu symptoms such as chilliness, abundant clear urination, diarrhea, and urinary incontinence.  Mingmen fortifies a tired condition and lack of vitality; it alleviates depression, weak knees, and weak legs.  It may be indicated by a pale tongue and a deep, weak pulse.

Mingmen benefits the yang aspect of the Kidney

essence and is indicated in all sexual disorders from weakness of essence evidenced by impotence, premature ejaculation, nocturnal emission, and bone disorders. It strengthens the low back and knees, expels cold, and dries damp-cold, especially with the use of moxa. However, we need to be careful because moxa is very warming and can cause heat aggravation, particularly if there are also signs of Kidney yin xu. Discontinue moxa if signs of heat aggravation develop. Other conditions that can be treated include leukorrhea, diarrhea, profuse clear urination, abdominal, and uterine pain.

Mingmen calms the spirit, benefits and clears the brain. It treats seizures, mania, meningitis, disorientation, forgetfulness, fear, fright, insomnia, and dizziness.

Dachangshu, BL 25, is the Back Shu point of the Large Intestine. Remembering the clinical utility of Back Shu points, which are indicated to adjust qi and blood, BL 25 eliminates stagnation of qi and blood of the intestines that may cause pain, numbness, muscular atrophy, and motor impairment of the back and lower extremities. Dachangshu promotes the function of the Large Intestine and removes obstructions from the channel. It regulates the Large Intestine and Stomach, reducing constipation or diarrhea, dysentery, painful defecation or urination, abdominal distention, and intestinal noise. It benefits low back pain or strain, pain in the sacroiliac joint, and relieves fullness, swelling, and paralysis of the lower extremities.

Yaoyangguan, GV 3, tonifies Kidney yang and qi. As such, it strengthens the lower back and legs. It is beneficial for irregular menstruation, nocturnal emission, and impotence. Very frequently used as a local point for backaches, particularly from Kidney yang deficiency, it is indicated especially when the backache radiates to the legs. It is beneficial for pain in the lumbosacral region, numbness, muscular atrophy, motor impairment, weakness of the legs, and knee pain caused by Kidney qi and yang xu.  With moxa it warms cold and dries damp-cold that may produce leukorrhea, diarrhea, colitis, and lower abdominal distention.

Bladder 40 (Weizhong) is the he (sea) point of the Bladder channel.  Elementally, it is the earth point and the controlling point of that channel.  As such, it is very effective in clearing and resolving heat and dampness from the Bladder and Intestines that causes burning urination, ulcerations, diarrhea, and urinary incontinence.  It clears summer-heat in acute attacks of heat in the summertime that manifest as burning fever, delirium, skin rashes, and unconsciousness from heatstroke.  It cools the blood and drains heat from the blood especially with bloodletting technique.  Thus, it clears skin diseases, carbuncles, boils, herpes, fever, malarial disorders, restless fetus disorders, and epistaxis.

BL 40 eliminates blood stasis and channel obstructions that create lower leg or abdominal pain.  Weizhong relaxes the sinews and tendons, opens the channel to benefit the lower back, knees, hips, and legs.  Although the use of this point is very good for chronic or acute, excess or deficiency type backaches, it is most effective for acute and excess varieties, especially when the backache is either bilateral or unilateral, not on the midline.  Lower back pain, sciatica, hip joint pain, restricted movement, lower extremity paralysis, all knee joint diseases, gastrocnemius muscle spasms, convulsions, and muscular tetany can be treated through this point.

As in all cases of tonification and dispersion, needle retention times are relative and will vary.  As a general rule, however, needles should be retained for approximately twenty minutes.  The needle retention is able to strengthen and deepen the stimulation of the techniques to give greatest effect.  Although the overall effect of the treatment is tonification of Kidney qi and yang, the technique applied to each set of points depends on whether the point needs to be tonified or dispersed. This decision can be made by properly discerning the pathology of each point.

In conclusion, if the practitioner has secured the correct differentiation of the back pain so that it matches the criteria of Eight Needle Technique, results are swift, efficacious, and long lasting, often with added benefits from tonifying Kidney qi and yang xu as *Case 7* notes.

**Case 7.** Eight Needle Technique for back pain and overall tonification.

The patient was a thirty-five-year-old woman with a history of chronic lower back problems due to trauma. She also had many signs and symptoms of Kidney qi and yang xu such as cold hands and feet, lethargy, problems with memory and concentration, weak legs, blurred vision, irregular, scanty menses, and dizziness. She had received acupuncture for this problem and experienced good to fair results. Scalp acupuncture in particular helped her significantly.

She received an Eight Needle treatment by a student practitioner just learning the technique. The point locations should have been more accurate and the depths of needle insertions should have been deeper. Though the qi was grasped, the tonification technique was weak. In spite of these areas that could have been improved, the patient still reported that during the treatment her back pain diminished. Several days later her back still felt good, though not perfect. However, she was pleasantly surprised to find that in general she felt better: more energetic and more alert. Her legs were stronger, her eyes brighter, and her head felt less empty. This is a good example of the local and systemic effects of Eight Needle Technique.

# TEN NEEDLE TECHNIQUE

I n chronic conditions, when deficiency of qi, blood, or yin is the primary diagnosis, the "Ten Needle Technique" treatment can be used either as a treatment plan in and of itself or as the skeletal formula to which other points are added based on signs and symptoms. This formula can be applied in a variety of clinical situations. It is obvious in clinical practice that deficiency of the essential substances of qi, blood, and yin are not only commonly encountered but are difficult to treat because they indicate long-term, chronic conditions. Interestingly, I have found this treatment approach to be effective in tonifying yang as well. Thus, this formula can tonify qi, blood, yin, *and* yang, certainly an efficient prescription.

*Table 22* summarizes the points used in Ten Needle Technique, their locations, angles, and insertion depths. A discussion of the primary energetics that account for the utility of this valuable formula follows. A note of caution should be observed concerning the insertion depths of these needles, which are the recommended depths from Chinese texts. As always, these depths are a range and should be adjusted according to the patient's presentation, since many patients are thin, guarded, or vulnerable in the abdominal region and along the Conception Vessel.

*Table 22.* Ten Needle Technique: Points, Locations, Angles, and Depths of Insertions

| Points | Locations | Angles and Depths of Insertions |
| --- | --- | --- |
| CV 13 (Shangguan) | On the midline of the abdomen, 5 cun above the center of the umbilicus | Perpendicular .5 in.–1.2 in. |
| CV 12 (Zhongwan) | On the midline of the abdomen, 4 cun above the center of the umbilicus | Perpendicular .5 in.–1.2 in. |
| CV 10 (Xiawan) | On the midline of the abdomen, 2 cun above the center of the umbilicus | Perpendicular .5 in.–1.2 in. |
| ST 25 (Tianshu) (bilateral) | 2 cun lateral to the center of the umbilicus | Perpendicular .7 in.–1.2 in.<br><br>The moxa box can be added from CV 10 to ST 25 and below to tonify yang |
| ST 36 (Zusanli) (bilateral) | 3 cun below ST 35, 1 finger breath lateral to the anterior crest of the tibia | Perpendicular .5 in.–1.2 in. |
| CV 6 (Qihai) | On the midline of the abdomen, 1.5 cun below the umbilicus | Perpendicular .8 in.–1.2 in. |
| PC 6 (Neiguan) (bilateral) | 2 cun above the wrist crease, between the tendons of the muscles palmaris longus and flexor carpi radialis | Perpendicular .5 in.–.8 in. |

# Clinical energetics of the points

## CV 13 (Shangguan)

This point controls the upper orifice of the Stomach (cardiac sphincter) so that food can enter the Stomach to begin the rotting and ripening process. In this way qi, blood, and yin are produced and Stomach qi descends more fully.

## CV 12 (Zhongwan)

CV 12 combined with CV 13 raises the yang and sinking Spleen qi.

CV 12, the Front Mu point of the Stomach, is one of the Eight Influential points that dominates the fu organs. As such, it is involved in receiving, digesting, absorbing, transmitting, and excreting food. It regulates Stomach qi and tonifies chronic Spleen and Stomach problems such as deficiency of qi, yin, or yang. It also resolves dampness.

As an important vortex—a crossing point of many meridians—CV 12 is a very powerful point. The following energies center around it:

a. The internal pathway of the Lung meridian begins at CV 12.
b. The Spleen, Heart, and Small Intestine meridians pass through Zhongwan.
c. The Liver meridian ends there.
d. The Large Intestine and Triple Warmer meridians begin there.
e. The point is located along the Ren channel pathway.
f. Located at the midpoint of the Stomach, the point controls the middle of the Stomach, tonifying the Spleen and Stomach so they can produce qi, blood, and yin and resolve dampness. It regulates Stomach qi and is useful for chronic Stomach and Spleen problems. It suppresses rebellious Stomach qi and is good for neurasthenia and emotional problems.

## CV 10 (Xiawan)

Xiawan controls the lower orifice of the Stomach (pylorus), encouraging Stomach qi to descend. It relieves food stagnation and tonifies the Spleen and Stomach so that food is broken down and transformed into qi, blood, or yin. Because of its lower location in relation to the Stomach, it is helpful in resolving indigestion, stomachache, prolapse of the stomach, diarrhea, and acute stomach problems.

## ST 25 (Tianshu)

As the Front Mu point of the Large Intestine, according to the *Neijing (The Yellow Emperor's Classic),* ST 25 adjusts the intestines in any condition, that is, it clears heat, regulates qi, relieves food retention, and eliminates stagnation.

According to the *Nanjing (The Classic of Difficult Questions),* Stomach 25 is the Front Mu point of the Lungs, hence the condition of the lungs can be determined at ST 25 on the right side of the body. According to Yoshio Manaka,[1] ST 25 is the Front Mu point of the Triple Warmer on the right side of the body (the explanation for this is too complex to discuss here and will be found in my forthcoming book, "The Magic Hand Returns Spring, The Art of Palpatory Diagnosis").

On the left, ST 25 is an extremely reliable indicator of blood stagnation and Liver blood stagnation in particular. The reason for this is that at the site of ST 25 on the left, the portal vein, which carries nutrients to the liver to be packaged into packets of glycogen or stored energy, exits from the large intestine and goes to the liver. As a result, when Liver qi is stagnant, it frequently leads to Liver blood stagnation and manifests at ST 25 on the left because of this liver-large intestine connection. Correspondingly, when there is a blockage at Stomach 25 on the left, it can cause Liver qi stagnation. When this point is not blocked and is free-flowing, it opens the lower warmer (jiao) and the channels to nourish the qi of the lower jiao. It is a storehouse of energy.

## ST 36 (Zusanli)

Zusanli opens the lower warmer, regulates the intestines, and builds Kidney yin. It brings energy down.

It benefits and regulates the Stomach and Spleen, controlling the epigastric area. As the lower he (sea) point, ST 36 sends a vessel directly to the Stomach.

As the horary point on an earth meridian, ST 36

---

1 See Kiiko Matsumoto, *Hara Diagnosis, Reflections on the Sea.* Paradigm Publications, Brookline, Mass., 1988; p 350.

tonifies and adjusts the qi and blood of the whole body. It stimulates qi production and dispels cold. It strengthens the body's resistance, increases immunity, and strengthens the antipathogenic factor. It regulates yin and wei qi. It raises the yang and strengthens weak and deficient conditions.

### CV 6 (Qihai)

This point is at the center of the vital energy in the body, the Dan Tian, where the living qi of the Kidney resides. It is useful for all states of exhaustion and insufficiency. Especially with the use of moxa, it tonifies qi, yang, and yin; regulates qi; tonifies original qi; resolves damp; augments Kidney deficiency; and strengthens the will to live.

### PC 6 (Neiguan)

Neiguan assists in communication between and treatment of the three jiaos; it keeps qi and blood flowing in their proper pathways.

As Master of the Yinwei Mai, it measures and/or produces yin defensive energy.

Coupled with the Spleen meridian and the Chong Mai vessel, PC 6 assists Spleen and Kidney functions. *(See Chapter Fourteen for a full discussion of PC 6.)*

## Applications

An example of using Ten Needle Technique in combination with other points would be to add CV 3 (Zhongji), Front Mu point of the Bladder, and SP 6 (Sanyinjiao), Group Luo of the Three Leg Yin, for cases of urinary retention. Add a moxa box for greater therapeutic results as long as there are no signs of heat.

It is apparent from an analysis of the formula that Ten Needle Technique is a beneficial formula to employ when there are many symptoms pointing in the direction of deficiency.  But sometimes very deficient patients whom this formula would benefit cannot tolerate the insertion of ten needles, in which case the following modifications can be made:

1. Needle PC 6 (Neiguan) only on the left side because Pericardium energetics are more left sided.  (There is a discussion of the theoretical justification for this fact in Chapter Fourteen ).

2. Pretest by palpating Conception Vessel 13 (Shangguan), CV 12 (Zhongwan) and CV 10 (Xiawan) and select the most tender point to needle.

3. As "Heaven's Pivot," ST 25 (Tianshu) should always be needled bilaterally to establish an equilibrium between qi and blood.  As I discussed previously under the energetics of that point, ST 25 on the right side is a qi reflex point and ST 25 on the left is a blood stagnation point.  Needling both points helps to balance qi and blood.

4. CV 6 (Qihai) must always be included in this strategy.

5. ST 36 (Zusanli) can be needled only on the right side due to the affinity of Stomach energetics for the right.

These modifications can be effective especially if the practitioner's tonification needle technique is proficient enough to compensate for the reduced number of needles.

If no signs of heat are present (either of the excess or deficient type) the addition of the moxa box is incomparable, particularly for tonifying the yang.  Carefully position the moxa box over the lower abdomen with the upper border of the box just above the navel, close to the CV 10 (Xiawan)–CV 9 (Shuifen) area.  The lower border should be on the abdomen so that it covers CV 6 (Qihai) and ST 25 (Tianshu) as well (see *Figure 12* for correct moxa box positioning).  Ignite two three-inch pieces of moxa stick at both ends and allow them to burn for ten to twenty minutes.  Exercise caution with patients who have neurological disorders that produce a lack of sensitivity to pain, elderly patients, others with delicate skin, or those who have not had their abdomen, and especially the navel, recently exposed to sun. The first time the box is used, the retention time should be short until the practitioner is sure that the patient can tolerate the heat.   For the first few treatments, monitor the patient's reactions by checking the patient's skin under the box at periodic intervals.

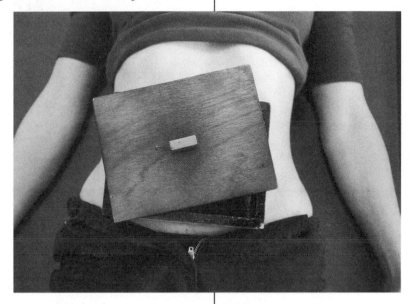

***Figure 12.*** Moxa Box Positioning

After the administration of the Ten Needle Technique, patients generally will not experience a great surge of energy, but rather a deep-seated feeling of relaxation and perhaps even tiredness as the energy being tonified consolidates itself on a very deep level. Patients should be advised of this therapeutic reaction so they know what to expect.  Ten Needle Technique can be administered as a course of treatment (that is, ten consecutive treatments) or as a periodic tonification treatment.

*Case 8* describes a rather interesting clinical application of this treatment protocol in the treatment of emotions.

**Case 8.** The application of Ten Needle Technique in the treatment of emotions

The patient was a thirty-five-year-old female with no real physical complaint. She had made an appointment with me for "a tune-up." As a victim of incest, her most long-standing problem was mastering her emotions. She also had lots of stress at work, and she was very high-strung.

In answer to the Ten Questions, the subpathologies included gas, over-thinking, waking up at night, a heavy period, abdominal distention, feeling hot, ravenous appetite, some facial breakouts, feeling tight in the intestines, hip joint pain, nighttime urination, exhaustion from time to time, pinpoint pain in the heart, and occasional vaginal discharge.

She had no Western medical diagnosis and she was taking no medication or treatment for these symptoms which she did not view as significant or problematic. The tongue was reddish-purple, with a red tip and small yin xu cracks developing. The surface was rough and had no coating except for a greasy one in the lower jiao. The pulse on the left side was thin and weak in all positions. On the right it was stronger but more superficial and slippery. The most significant palpatory finding was a shallow, tight, hard stomach at CV 12.

Fifteen treatments constituted the course of therapy needed for both the practitioner and the patient to feel that she was balanced. At that point, every subpathology listed above was resolved and the patient felt better emotionally. She wanted to be balanced and wanted to learn how to deal with her emotions better. She relied upon the practitioner to educate her about what the subpathologies were and what their significance was. When the abdomen started clearing, the symptoms started to resolve quickly. When CV 12, the Front Mu of the Stomach, the source of all yin, was no longer tender, the patient reported feeling warm, nurtured, and taken care of. Prior to one of the last treatments, she had an abnormal uterine bleeding at ovulation after which she felt a "new freedom in her abdomen."

The Ten Needle Technique, preceded by "abdominal clearing,"[2] was the primary modality employed, although herbs were also prescribed to supplement the treatment. The patient was very receptive to deep breathing, awareness of body energetics, patient education, and compliance with herbs. She felt that all these modalities had given her the tools to cope better.

---

2. "Abdominal clearing" is a Japanese treatment technique. Japanese acupuncture is the theme of my next book, "The Magic Hand Returns Spring, The Art of Palpatory Diagnosis," forthcoming in 1997.

# CHAPTER 11

# THE EIGHT CURIOUS VESSELS IN ORIENTAL MEDICINE

## General Functions

The Eight Curious Vessels in Oriental medicine are interesting for the serious student of Eastern medicine who seeks to understand more about bodily energetics and meridian function. Apart from some esoteric literature, the Eight Curious Vessels (or the Eight Extra or Extraordinary Meridians) are only superficially understood and used. The purpose of this discussion is to provide the practitioner with a viable, working body of knowledge on this large and important topic.

Nguyen Van Nghi, M.D., the well-known European classical acupuncturist, says that the subject is "not a small idea"[1] and the discussion in this book is by no means complete. He suggests, as do I, that these vessels are tools for thinking about bodily energetics. The Eight Extraordinary Meridians are presented here for the practitioner with this approach in mind. Thus, when we use them, we are not treating diseases as much as differentiating syndrome paradigms. These are patterns of interaction between the twelve main meridians and other meridian systems. Hence the pathology of a "Curious Vessel" is characterized by symptoms that encompass several channels.

A search of the available literature reveals that the

1. Van Nghi N: An exploration of the eight curious vessels. Lecture, Southwest Acupuncture College, Santa Fe, N.M., Sept., 1987.

way the Eight Extraordinary Meridians are used varies somewhat according to the Chinese, European, and Japanese approaches, the cultures that have explored them most intensely. It is my intention to put their crucial functions in the human body into easily understandable terms so beginning students of acupuncture, as well as experienced practitioners, can use these meridians in their practices.

As practitioners know, they are called by various names: the Eight Extra Meridians, the Eight Extraordinary Meridians, the Eight Secondary Vessels, the Eight Miscellaneous Meridians, and the Eight Psychic Channels. Dr. Van Nghi summarizes their functions in the body and claims that they are not extra, extraordinary, or secondary. Whereas the twelve main meridians may be easier to understand because they have a somewhat Western counterpart (that is, an associated organ), Dr. Van Nghi suggests that the functions of these vessels are indeed curious, and hence he prefers to call them the Eight Curious Vessels.

In terms of clinical usage, the Eight Curious Vessels have nine major functions. These functions cover a broad range of disorders that are difficult to treat and hence may require subtle and novel treatment strategies. The Curious Vessels are particularly well-suited for these specific disharmonies whose resolution can be more rapid by using them. The nine functions are discussed below and summarized in *Table 23*.

## 1. Homeostatic

The Eight Curious Vessels have a unique capacity as homeostatic vessels. For example, they can absorb excess perverse energy from the twelve main meridians. The perverse energy may be an exogenous, endogenous, or miscellaneous pathogen or a secondary pathological product. By combining the Master and Coupled points of each set of paired meridians, the Curious Vessels are able to drain or sap these pathogens with remarkable ease. For example SI 3 (Houxi) and BL 62 (Shenmai) plus points along the Governing Vessel Channel can be used to treat intermittent fevers caused by an invasion of an exogenous pathogen.

*Table 23.* An Orientation to the Clinical Functions of the Eight Curious Vessels

| FUNCTION | | USE |
|---|---|---|
| Homeostatic | Absorbs excess perverse energy from the twelve main meridians | To treat fever caused by invasion of an exogenous pathogen |
| Circulatory | Warms and defends the surface by circulating wei qi | To increase yang in body |
| Enriching | Enriches the body with qi, blood, and ancestral qI | To treat deficiencies in those areas |
| Controlling | Serves as reservoirs and conductors of jing | To treat essence deficiency illness and the developmental life cycle |
| Nourishing | Harmonizes and nourishes the blood vessels, bone, brain, Gall Bladder, uterus, and bone marrow | To treat diseases of the Liver, Gall Bladder, uterus, brain |
| Supervisory | Exerts a commanding role over areas of the body, essential substances and zang-fu organs | To treat zones of the body, essential substances, and zang-fu organs |
| Balancing | Regulates energy | When the pulses are balanced but the patient still complains of symptoms |
| | | When the twelve main meridians have failed, and to treat the root causes of a disease |
| Supplementing | Supplements multiple deficiencies | To treat chronic disease, metabolic and hormonal disorders, psychic strain |
| Adjusting | Reduces inherited or acquired structural stress | To treat muscle tension, postural or structural stress |

## 2. Circulatory

Another relationship that the Curious Vessels have with exogenous pathogens is that because the Curious Meridians circulate wei qi, which warms and defends the surface, they can protect the body from outside invasion. As the "General who Governs the Yang" the Governing Vessel Channel has the particular but not exclusive function of increasing wei qi.

## 3. Enriching

The Curious Vessels, however, are not only adept at

annihilating perverse exogenous energy, they are also able to supply deficiencies and enrich the body with qi, blood, and ancestral qi when the body is weak. As early, structural, formative energies, rich in qi and blood, they are able to do this. They are the internal dynamic of development.

## 4. Controlling

In 1985, the World Health Organization agreed that all the Eight Curious Vessels originate in the Kidney. Thus, the Kidney plays an important role in controlling the development of the body, which it regulates.[2] As a result, the Kidney assumes an important role in controlling the stages of both male and female life cycles. *Table 24* summarizes the origins of the Eight Curious Vessels, the conventional thought on their origins.

*Table 24.* Origins of the Eight Curious Vessels

| MERIDIAN | ORIGIN |
| --- | --- |
| Du | Inside of lower abdomen |
| Ren | Lower abdomen, uterus |
| Chong | Uterus, lower abdomen |
| Dai | Below the hypochondrium |
| Yinqiao | Posterior aspect of the navicular bone |
| Yangqiao | Lateral side of the heel |
| Yinwei | Medial side of the leg |
| Yangwei | Heel |

Many Kidney disorders pertain to the female life cycle of growth, development, and decline and consequently fall within the domain of problems that the Curious Meridians are particularly good at dealing with. Using the Curious Vessels in this manner allows the practitioner to effectively treat the physiology and pathology of women.

Consequently, the Curious Vessels are rich reservoirs

---

2. The World Health Organization is standardizing acupuncture nomenclature. Further information can be obtained from The World Health Organization, Regional Office for the Western Pacific, P.O. Box 2932, Manila, Philippines.

and conductors of jing, the quintessence of energy. As sources of prenatal and postnatal qi, they can supplement the body's energy, making them particularly effective meridians for the treatment of "essence deficiency" diseases, that is, chronic debilitating illnesses such as early aging, menopause, multiple sclerosis, chronic fatigue, and AIDS.

## 5. Nourishing

As conductors of jing, the Eight Curious Vessels nourish the ancestral, extraordinary organs—the blood vessels, bone, brain, Gall Bladder, uterus, and bone marrow. Nourishment of the uterus makes childbearing possible. The Curious Vessels nourish the arteries and circulatory system, the brain, the bones, and marrow, and they harmonize the Liver and Gall Bladder. Diseases of any of these organs (Liver, Gall Bladder, uterus, or brain) or systems (hepatobiliary, circulatory, skeletal) can be uniquely treated through the Curious Vessels.

## 6. Supervisory

The Curious Vessels energetically relate to both the organs and the meridians because they intersect with the twelve main meridians. Because of this connection, they reinforce the points of the twelve regular channels and harmonize the zones between the principal meridians. They thus command or supervise various parts of the body and its functions. For example, the Governing Channel supervises the qi of the primary yang channels and has a strong influence on the Liver, brain, and Kidneys. *Table 25* illustrates in summary form the physiological functions and physical zones and meridian symptomatology of the Eight Curious Vessels.

*Table 25.* The Eight Curious Vessels: Portion of the Body Governed, Physiological Function, and Channel Pathology

| MERIDIAN | PORTION OF THE BODY GOVERNED | PHYSIOLOGICAL FUNCTION | CHANNEL PATHOLOGY |
|---|---|---|---|
| Du | Neck, shoulders, back, inner canthus | Regulates and stimulates yang energy, increases wei qi, and circulates the yang of the whole body; for attack by pathogens, particularly wind-cold at the Taiyang stage. Supervises the qi of the yang channels. Has a strong influence on the Liver. Nourishes the brain, Kidneys, spinal cord. Tends to absorb excess energy from the yang meridians above GV 14 and supply energy to them when they are deficient below GV 14 | Stiffness and pain in spinal column, headache, epilepsy, opisthotonos, diseases of the CNS, intermittent fever, yang mental illness (hallucinations), cold, numb extremities, insufficiency of wei qi |
| Ren | Throat, chest, lungs, epigastric region | Concentration of yin energy, controls all the yin meridians. Nourishes the uterus. Absorbs excess energy from yin meridians below CV 8 and supplies energy if they are deficient above CV 8. For yin and blood problems. Commands diseases related to blood and gynecology | Leukorrhea, irregular menses, hernia, retention of urine, pain in the epigastric region and lower abdomen, infertility in both men and women, nocturnal emission, enuresis, pain in the genitals, rebellious qi in the chest, hormonal problems during menopause and puberty due to stagnation of qi and blood, dysmenorrhea, fibroids, cysts, hot blood problems, chronic itching, pharyngitis, heart disease, stagnation of the whole genital system, genital problems due to stagnation of qi and blood |
| Chong | Heart, chest, lungs | Arouses Three Leg Yin (SP, KI, LR) | Spasm and pain in the abdomen, irregular menstruation, infertility in men and women, asthmatic breathing, removes obstructions and masses, circulates blood, regulates life cycle changes, hormonal sensitivity of uterus, weak digestion from poor constitution with damp-phlegm accumulation, menstrual problems related to Spleen, stagnation and obstruction |
| Dai | Retroauricular region cheek, outer canthus, mastoid region | Promotes pelvic/leg circulation, nourishes hepatobiliary system, supplies deficiencies, influences downward flow of energy. Its disturbances always affect meridians that it encircles at the level of the waist, i.e., SP, ST, KI, Chong, GV, CV. Its energy depends upon the Yangming and GB being sufficient, otherwise the Dai is not nourished, leading to pain, paralysis, and so on. Controls circulation at the waist and downward | Abdominal pain, weakness and pain of the lumbar area, leukorrhea, hip problems, irregular menses, distention and fullness in the abdomen, prolapse of uterus, muscular atrophy, motor impairment of lower extremities, migraines |
| Yinqiao | Lower abdomen, lumbar and hip area, pubis | Brings fluid and jing to the eyes; secondary vessel of the Kidney | Hypersomnia, yin xu especially at night, spasm of lower limbs, inversion of foot, epilepsy, lethargy, pain in the lower abdomen, pain in the lumbar region and hip referring to the pubis, problems of eyes, genitals, bone marrow, genital stagnation; used mainly for women |
| Yangqiao | Inner canthus, back, lumbar region, lower limbs | Secondary vessel to Bladder, absorbs excess energy of head (brain, eyes) | Epilepsy, insomnia, redness and pain of inner canthus, pain in back, lumbar region, eversion of foot, spasms of lower limbs |
| Yinwei | Interior syndromes | Preserver of the yin; principal vessel of the Kidney; binds the yin | Cardialgia, chest pain, all yin xu especially of the heart |
| Yangwei | Exterior syndromes | Preserver of the yang; binds all yang meridians | Chills and fever, imbalance in defensive energy |

## 7. Balancing

Because of the energetic relationships between the organs and all of the meridians, the use of the Eight Curious Vessels facilitates treatment of the root cause of a disease regardless of its etiology, therefore the Eight Curious Vessels can be used when the twelve main meridians have failed.

As the precursors to the twelve main meridians, the Curious Vessels regulate the qi and blood of the main meridians. Therefore, the Eight Curious Vessels can be used when the pulses are balanced but the patient still complains of symptoms. In this case, the patient's signs and symptoms must correspond to Eight Curious Vessel pathology (see *Table 25*).

## 8. Supplementing

When a multiplicity of deficiencies points in the same direction (for example, generalized yin xu, yang xu, or specific organ deficiency such as Kidney qi xu, and so on) the Eight Curious Vessels may be employed. Other examples include chronic disease, depleted energy, metabolic and hormonal disorders, mental/psychological strain, or when too many needles would weaken the patient.

## 9. Adjusting

For palpable or spontaneous muscle tension and postural or structural stress that is either inherited or acquired, the Eight Curious Meridians are particularly well-suited because they are the residue of the earliest formative energies created just after conception. They are the first primordial meridians, the outlines of who we are and what we may become. Their existence predates the zang-fu, the tendinomuscular meridians, the Luo, and the divergent meridians. They are the fundamental source of our body armor as well as the genetic basis of who we are and how we may develop.

*Taiyang and Yang Ming as used in Table 25 are stages in the "Six Divisions," a theoretical framework described in the Shang Han Lun (Treatise of Cold-Induced Disorders). The Six Divisions explain the penetration of a cold or wind-cold pathogen into the body and how the symptoms change as the pathogen penetrates more deeply. For a succinct and useful summary of the Six Divisions, see Kaptchuk T: The Web That Has No Weaver. Congdon and Weed, New York, 1983; pp 269–271 and Maciocia G: Tongue Diagnosis in Chinese Medicine. Eastland Press, Seattle, 1995, pp 173-185.*

As such, they are particularly beneficial in the treatment of both inherited as well as acquired musculoskeletal disorders.

*Table 26* offers a unique view on how to use these vessels by looking at an interpretation of their Chinese characters (keep in mind that Chinese characters are not static but energetic symbols and have many meanings). This vision offered by Kiiko Matsumoto provides valuable insight into their clinical use.[4] Finally, *Table 27* gives a summary of the Eight Curious Vessels, their significant points, and treatment approaches.

In conclusion, these charts give practitioners an "idea," an orientation, of how to use the Eight Curious Vessels based on the following:

a. the meaning of the vessel's name, for example, "Governs all the yang" (*Tables 26* and *27*)

b. the portion of the body governed, both internal and external pathways, for example, "neck, shoulders, back" (*Table 25*)

c. physiological function, for example, "increases circulation of wei qi" (*Table 25*), and

d. indications, for example, "intermittent fever, cold" (*Table 25*)

*Table 26.* Additional Meanings of the Names of the Curious Vessels

| MERIDIAN | NAME |
|---|---|
| Du | *General who governs Yang.* The sea of various yang chings. |
| Ren | *Pregnancy, obligation.* To accept or hold something in front of the abdomen. The sea of yin meridians. |
| Chong | *Street.* Used to express the idea of passing or transformation, alchemical transformation, two entities clashing together to produce something different. Assault, what goes up. |
| Dai | *Belt.* It that acts as support, bundles all the meridians together. |
| Wei | *Rope tied around something.* It pulls down and secures. Controls downward movement. Preserver of yin or yang, particularly yin and yang defensive energy. |

4. Matsumoto K: *Extraordinary Vessels.* Paradigm Publications, Brookline, Mass., 1986; p 3.

*Table 27.* A Summary of the Eight Curious Vessels: Significant Points and Treatment Approaches[5]

| MERIDIAN | MEANING OF NAME | MASTER POINTS | COUPLED POINTS | XI (CLEFT)/ LUO POINTS* | COALESCENT POINTS |
|---|---|---|---|---|---|
| DU MAI (GV) | Governor vessel. Governs all yang channels. | SI 3 | BL 62 | GV 1* | X |
| REN MAI (CV) | Conception vessel. Responsible to all yin channels and nourishes the fetus. | LU 7 | KI 6 | CV 15* | X |
| CHONG MAI (TV) | Sea of Blood, Sea of Arteries and Meridians, Thoroughfare Vessel, Penetrating Vessel. Vital channel communicating with all the channels; regulates the qi and blood of the twelve regular meridians. | SP 4 | PC 6 | X | CV 1, KI 11-21 |
| DAI MAI (DV) | Belt Vessel, Girdle Channel. Binds all the channels. | GB 41 | TE 5 | X | GB 26, 27, 28 |
| YINQIAO MAI (YINHV) | Yin Heel Vessel, Heel agility, Accelerator of the yin. | KI 6 | LU 7 | KI 8 | KI 6, 8 |
| YANGQIAO MAI (YANGHV) | Yang Heel Vessel, Accelerator of the yang. | BL 62 | SI 3 | BL 59 | BL 1, 59, 61, 62, GB 20, 29, SI 10, ST 4, 3, 1, LI 15, 16 |
| YINWEI MAI (YINLV) | Yin Link Vessel, Connects with all yin channels. | PC 6 | SP 4 | KI 9 | KI 9, SP 13, 15, 16, LR 14, CV 22, 23 |
| YANGWEI MAI (YANGLV) | Yang Link Vessel, Connects with all yang channels. | TE 5 | GB 41 | GB 35 | BL 63, GB 35, 13-21, GV 15, 16, ST 8, SI 10, TE 15 |

# Applications of the Eight Curious Vessels, Jing Treatments

As I have said before, one important use of the Eight Curious Vessels is when a number of deficiencies point in the same direction. As practitioners of Chinese medicine are aware, deficiency is a common clinical experience. New types of illness characterized as "essence deficiency" diseases are becoming more common—from environmental contamination and cultural stress. When a patient presents with multiple deficiencies, it is often difficult to decide where to begin to treat. Also, these people rarely tolerate many needles. Multiple deficiencies often present as chronic fatigue, fibromyalgia, AIDS, multiple sclerosis, among others,

*Mai (sometimes transliterated as mo) means "channel or vessel."*

*Coalescent points: points of intersection between the twelve regular channels and the Eight Curious Vessels. Sources differ about the Coalescent points.*

*Confluent points: the Master points that connect the Eight Curious Vessels with the twelve regular meridians and activate the Curious Vessel.*

*This table uses World Health Organization standard nomenclature of the Curious Vessels and regular meridians.*

---

5. This chart is based on *Essentials of Chinese Acupuncture,* compiled by Beijing College of Traditional Chinese Medicine, Foreign Language Press, Beijing, PRC, 1980; pp 282–286.

and the jing treatment can be beneficial.

The jing treatment consists of needling the Eight Confluent points, that is, the Master points of the Eight Curious Vessels and CV 6 (Qihai). Needles are inserted from top to bottom beginning with the Master point of one meridian and its corresponding coupled meridian. I prefer to open the Dai meridian first as it is the only horizontal meridian and as such functionally binds all the twelve main meridians and the remaining Curious Vessels together. If the Dai meridian is obstructed, it can bind the other meridians in a dysfunctional manner and hence it is useful to open it at the start of treatment. (Dai meridian obstructions can develop from poor posture, excess weight, organ prolapses, tight clothing, pregnancy, and wearing high heels.) This is accomplished by needling TE 5 (Waiguan), usually on the right side, and then complementing this point by needling its Coupled point, GB 41 (Zulinqi), on the left.[6]

Next, I highly recommend needling PC 6 (Neiguan) on the left as a primary point to move any stagnation.[7] I believe that stagnation should be relieved before deficiencies are tonified so that any zonal blockages are not correspondingly or inadvertently tonified, that is, strengthened or exacerbated. SP 4 (Gongsun), the Coupled point, is subsequently needled on the right side.

LU 7 (Lieque) on the right and KI 6 (Zhaohai) on the left are then needled, followed by SI 3 (Houxi) on the left and BL 62 (Shenmai) on the right. Finally, CV 6 (Qihai) is inserted.

Some practitioners have reported that the order of needle insertion is not critical to the effectiveness of treatment. Just as I have done, the practitioner is encouraged to monitor and evaluate clinical results for

---

6. Gardner-Abbate S: Assessing and treating Pericardium-6 (Neiguan): gate to internal well-being. *Amer J Acupun*, 1995; 23(2): 159–167.

7. Assessing and treating Pericardium-6, 164.

the benefit of the patient.  The protocol presented here is my preferred treatment strategy.

Excellent technique when inserting and manipulating the needle is imperative to avoid pain at these Command points, as well as to achieve the desired result.  Needles should be retained from ten to thirty minutes depending on the patient's condition.  Start with shorter time periods to assess how the patient reacts and then as the patient gets stronger, the needles can be retained for a longer time.

This treatment works on a very deep energetic level.  As a result, when being needled, it is not uncommon for the patient to experience a state of relaxation instead of being superficially energized.  Patients may desire to rest further after the treatment and they should be encouraged to wait until they feel ready before leaving the office.  In addition, they should be advised not to expend energy unnecessarily so that the vital qi contacted during the treatment is allowed to consolidate at a deeper level.

Sometimes practitioners are concerned that they should not use the Eight Curious Vessels at all or infrequently.  However, a review of their multiple and important functions, as well as clinical experience, does not discourage and in fact supports their careful use. *Table 28* summarizes the Eight Confluent point protocol in terms of point location, angle and depth of insertion, needling, and palpation technique.

*Table 28.* Eight Confluent Point Protocol

| POINT ORDER | EIGHT CURIOUS VESSEL MASTER POINT | COUPLED POINT | SIDE OF BODY TO PALPATE | PALPATION METHOD | SENSATION | POINT LOCATION | NEEDLE TECHNIQUE (JAPANESE NEEDLES BEST— #1G) |
|---|---|---|---|---|---|---|---|
| TE 5 (Waiguan) | Yangwei Mai | GB 41 (Zulinqi) | Right side | Deep palpation to PC 6, perpendicular pressure. Relatively speaking palpation on this side will be more shallow because yang side is more muscular and yin more mushy | Not as strong as subsequent points but when relevant, patient perceives sensation at the point | Standard TE 5 location | Perpendicular superficial insertion .3 in. No or small manipulation depending upon patient's constitution |
| GB 41 (Zulinqi) | Dai Mai | TE 5 (Waiguan) | Left side | Vigorous rubbing | Point is shallow and extremely painful in general | Two locations: standard GB 41 location and Japanese location in the depression anterior to the cuboid bone | For either location, obliquely .3 in. in the direction of the meridian (toward toe) |
| PC 6 (Neiguan) | Yinwei Mai | SP 4 (Gongsun) | Left side | Deep perpendicular palpation to TE 5 | Very tender when pathological | Standard PC 6 location | Superficial insertion .3 in. No or light manipulation depending upon patient's constitution |
| SP 4 (Gongsun) | Chong Mai | PC 6 (Neiguan) | Right side | Solid rub against the bone | Extremely painful in most cases | Standard SP 4 location | Perpendicular or oblique insertion .3 in. If oblique, needle in direction of meridian (toward heel) |
| LU 7 (Lieque) | Ren Mai | KI 6 (Zhaohai) | Right side | Push against bone | Not much comes up on palpation because of the size of the point but it can. Other signs and symptoms will support the use of the point | Standard LU 7 location | Obliquely .3 in. in direction of the meridian (toward thumb). Sometimes I go up the arm for dispersion |
| KI 6 (Zhaohai) | Yinqiao Mai | LU 7 (Lieque) | Both sides | With thumb push into the point | Characteristically tender, usually more on one side than another<br><br>Choose most tender | One of the alternate Chinese locations defined as 1 cun below medial malleolus, but slightly superior to the junction of the red and the white skin in a depression generally marked with a (X) fold in the skin | Posteriorly horizontally .1–2 in. in direction of meridian (toward heel) |
| SI 3 (Houxi) | Du Mai | BL 62 (Shenmai) | Left side | Obliquely upward against the bone | In terms of frequency does not come up that often, except when indicated and then there is some sensation that the patient reports | Standard SI 3 location | Perpendicular or obliquely upward (toward fingers) .2 in.–.3 in. |
| BL 62 (Shenmai) | Yangqiao Mai | SI 3 (Houxi) | Right side | This is a shallow point; firmly rub it | Generally very sore | Japanese BL 62 location which is closer to the Chinese BL 61 location | Obliquely .2 in.–.3 in. in the direction of the meridian (toward toes) |
| CV 6 (Qihai) | X | X | Center | In pathology, either a sensation of mushiness indicative of deficiency or hardness which is excess due to underlying deficiency. Resilient and good tone in health | Dislike if in pathology, sometimes invasive and guarded | On the midline of the abdomen 1.5 cun below the center of the umbilicus | Perpendicularly 1 in.–1.5 in. Summon qi to the area and tonify |

# CHAPTER 12

# THE CLINICAL SIGNIFICANCE
# OF THE CONFLUENT POINTS
## Applications in Gynecology

This chapter is devoted to the clinical significance of the Confluent points so that the practitioner can understand the unique energetics of each one. Because many of these functions have a positive effect on women's health, the application of these points to gynecological issues is stressed.

## 1. TE 5 (Waiguan)

The Luo point of the Triple Warmer meridian is TE 5 (Waiguan). It maintains the critical function of connecting all three jiaos, or burning spaces, where the essential substances—qi, blood, jing, and body fluid—are both created and harmoniously distributed to every part of the body for use or storage. Tenderness elicited at this point by palpation indicates problems with digestion. These problems can be stagnation from digestive pathology or the presence of the pathological by-products of phlegm, damp, and stagnant blood in one or more of the jiaos. Gynecological manifestations of these pathological by-products include leukorrhea, cysts, abdominal accumulations, and tumors of a benign or malignant nature.

*Wei* means "connection." TE 5 (Waiguan) as the Outer Gate, that is, as the Master of the Yangwei Mai (yang defensive system), mobilizes the yang defensive energies of the body. It connects all the yang channels that assist in protecting the organism. As Master point of the Yangwei Mai, Waiguan commands the outside of the body. Tenderness at this point may indicate a weakness in the yang organ-meridian systems or weakness in the true qi of the body that protects the person from outside evils. Thus, exterior syndromes are governed by TE 5 (Waiguan). Palpable tenderness at this site may indicate the tendency to be easily invaded by exogenous pathogens, which can further weaken the body's true qi because of the constant battle between the antipathogenic factor and the evil qi. It is a useful point for gynecological problems caused by exogenous invasion such as dysmenorrhea or leukorrhea.

## 2.  GB 41 (Zulinqi)

GB 41 (Zulinqi) is a primary point for women's health problems because of its intimate relationship to the Liver and the Dai channel. The Gall Bladder, as the yang functional counterpart of the Liver, can be viewed as an accurate index of Liver yang rising. In terms of gynecological function, this point is excruciatingly tender on palpation when the patient has Liver yang rising, because of Liver yin or blood deficiency, its most usual imbalance. Frequently, Kidney yin or qi xu is part of the scenario either as a causative factor or as a byproduct of Liver yin xu drawing from the Kidney. When GB 41 (Zulinqi) is tender, women are prone to scanty menses, cramps, breast tenderness, fibrocystic breasts, irritability, headache (migraine), or other PMS symptoms such as fatigue with the period, cravings for salt or other stimulants like chocolate, coffee, or spicy food that temporarily decongest Liver qi. Also, there can be mild back pain, constipation, and weakened vision.

GB 41 (Zulinqi) may also be sensitive if Liver qi is invading earth. As a result of wood overacting on earth, the Spleen qi usually becomes deficient. Damp accumulates and blood is not produced. Also, the Stomach can become hot as a result of this overacting cycle. Stomach yin is consumed and damp and phlegm develop. GB 41 (Zulinqi) is a yang point that can reflect the condition of the yin, particularly the yin deficiencies of the Liver, Kidney, and Stomach.

As the Horary point and wood point of the Gall Bladder meridian, GB 41 (Zulinqi) promotes the free flow of Liver qi. It is beneficial in resolving dampness in the genital region such as leukorrhea and in clearing phlegm-heat and stagnant blood that can cause symptoms of abdominal stagnation such as endometriosis and dysmenorrhea.

GB 41 (Zulinqi) is the Master point of the Dai channel, the one meridian that encircles, bundles, and ties the meridians together as the body's only horizontal support system. Its disturbances are harmful to the meridians it surrounds at the level of the waist (Gall Bladder, Spleen, Stomach, Kidney, Chong Mai, Conception Vessel, and Governing Vessel). Consequently, it regulates the jiaos above and below its pathway, influences leg and pelvic circulation, and contributes to the nourishment of the hepatobiliary system.

The health of the Dai channel depends on the ability of the Gall Bladder and Yangming (Stomach/Large Intestine) energy to create ample qi and blood. Gynecologically, the Dai Mai is implicated in irregular menses, leukorrhea, scanty menses, painful periods, and edema of the lower jiao.

Clinically, TE 5 (Waiguan) and GB 41 (Zulinqi) work synergistically. As depicted in *Figure 13*, the relationship between these two meridians (Yangwei Mai and

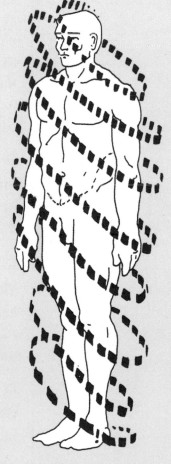

*Figure 13.* Image of the Functional Relationship between TE 5 (Waiguan) and GB 41 (Zulinqi)

Dai) can be compared to a spiral that encompasses all three jiaos longitudinally and latitudinally.

## 3.  PC 6 (Neiguan)

There is a complete discussion of this extremely important point in Chapter Fourteen, including references to gynecological health.  Here, I have simply listed the various energetic functions of Neiguan and have summarized each function briefly.

### A.  Neiguan as a Luo (Connecting) point

According to Chinese medicine, Luo points can be used as openings either to the transverse or to the longitudinal vessels.  As a transverse luo, a stimulus can be sent to the coupled organ-meridian complex—in this case, the San Jiao, the Triple Warmer.  Through the longitudinal luo, Neiguan stimulates its own organ-meridian complex through the internal pathway of the channel.

### B.  Neiguan as the Group Luo of the Three Arm Yin meridians

In this capacity, Neiguan binds together the Three Arm Yin meridians (the Lung, Heart, and Pericardium).

### C.  Neiguan as the Confluent (Master) Point of the Yinwei Mai

As the Confluent point of all the yin organ-meridian complexes (Lung, Heart, Pericardium, Liver, Spleen, and Kidney), Neiguan links them together.

### D.  Neiguan and Jueyin Energetic Level in the Six Divisions

In the Six Divisions, Neiguan is bound to the Liver at the Jueyin level.

### E.  Neiguan Coupled with the San Jiao in the Five Elements

The use of Neiguan to assess the immune function

derives from the fact that its connection to the Triple Warmer thereby connects it to the entire metabolism of the body.

### F. Pericardium-Uterus-Kidney Relationship

There is a connection from the Pericardium to the Kidney and from the Kidney to the uterus. This gives Neiguan considerable influence in gynecological issues. *(See Figure 16 in Chapter Fourteen.)*

### G. Coupled with the Chong Mai and its Confluent Point in the Eight Extra Vessel System

The Chong Mai and its Confluent (Master) point (SP 4, Gongsun) are coupled in the Eight Extra Vessel system with the Yinwei Mai.

### H. All the Eight Curious Vessels meet at PC 6 (Neiguan)

All the Eight Extra Meridians meet at Neiguan. This fact alone makes the point extremely important for the immune system and gynecological health.

## 4.  SP 4 (Gongsun)

Spleen 4 (Gongsun) is the Luo point of the Spleen organ-meridian complex. In this capacity, SP 4 (Gongsun) is useful in coordinating the functional relationship between the Spleen and the Stomach. It tonifies, pacifies, and regulates Spleen and Stomach disharmony, removes turbidity and obstruction, and circulates qi and blood. SP 4 (Gongsun) is useful in clearing obstructions of dampness from the Spleen, which can lead to cysts or leukorrhea. Additionally, it can quell fire in the Stomach that consumes yin and causes scanty menses, amenorrhea, and infertility.

Perhaps the most consistently painful point in the body, SP 4 (Gongsun) is exquisitely tender in patients with Spleen qi deficiency, damp accumulation, and blood deficiency patterns. These symptoms are characteristic of people who overwork, eat irregularly, worry excessively, or have poor nutritional patterns. Obviously, Spleen qi is essential for the sound energy of the entire body and gynecological health in particular because of its role in blood production and regulation. As a reactive point, SP 4 (Gongsun) can indicate blood deficiency manifesting as scanty menses or as PMS symptoms of headache, amenorrhea, backache, or dysmenorrhea from Liver qi stagnation arising out of blood deficiency.

Spleen 4 (Gongsun) is the Master point of the Chong meridian and the Coupled point of the Yinwei Mai. It is coupled energetically to PC 6 (Neiguan). The Chong meridian, translated variously as the "thoroughfare vessel," "the vital channel," "the sea of arteries and meridians," but more commonly known as the Sea of Blood, summarizes the role of the Chong as a reservoir of blood created by the joint efforts of the Spleen and Kidney. The Chong, like the Spleen and Kidney, flows upward, bringing with it the products of qi, blood, and body fluid. It regulates the qi and blood of the twelve regular channels and arouses the Three Leg Yin. As mentioned in the section on PC 6 (Neiguan), Gongsun and Neiguan work closely and homeostatically together to produce and distribute the basic body substances to every part of the body.

## 5. LU 7 (Lieque)

LU 7 (Lieque), the Luo connecting point of the Lung meridian, has the ability to tonify the qi of the Lungs and therefore of the whole body because the Lungs are the Master of the qi. As a Luo point, it sustains the energy of the whole body and is classically viewed as a general tonic point. It is also effective in dissipating water from the body. It stimulates its coupled organ, the Large Intestine, to do its job of being the Great

Eliminator. It removes the dregs that may deteriorate into pathological stagnation in the body. By virtue of its Luo point function and internal pathway the Lung meridian opens up the chest and sends its qi downward to be grasped by the Kidney. It is useful for rebellious qi in the chest, actually one of the best points. Dispersion of LU 7 (Lieque) as a Luo point will break up dampness or phlegm in the Lungs.

Lung 7 (Lieque) is the Master of the Ren Mai. Ren means responsibility and the Ren channel is responsible to all the yin channels. It is an extremely efficient point for opening the Ren channel so its energy can flow upward. LU 7 (Lieque) affects all the points on the Ren channel including the Mu points of the Pericardium, Heart, Stomach, Triple Burner, Kidney, Small Intestine, Bladder, and other points on the Ren channel that have important energetics. It passes through the uterus and nourishes the fetus. Gynecological problems from stagnant qi or blood—such as fibroids, painful periods, and cysts—are well treated with LU 7 (Lieque). The Ren channel is effective in absorbing excess energy from the yin meridians below CV 8 (Shenque) and can supply energy to the yin meridians if they are deficient above CV 8.

# 6. KI 6 (Zhaohai)

KI 6 (Zhaohai) is one of the most important points of the body, in some Japanese schools of thought perhaps *the* most important point. Its major function is to add yin to the body and it is generally considered the best point with which to nourish yin. It is extremely tender in patients with yin, or what could be termed preyin, deficiency. As a yin point, it is useful for cooling the blood and for promoting uterine and hormonal function. Zhaohai benefits the Kidney and strengthens vital essence.

One of the most common etiologies of jing and yin

deficiency is stress. KI 6 (Zhaohai) is considered to be the point that best indicates and treats Kidney yin xu. It is called the adrenal reflex point and denotes the effects of shock, trauma, chronic diseases, and lifestyle factors that have consumed yin.

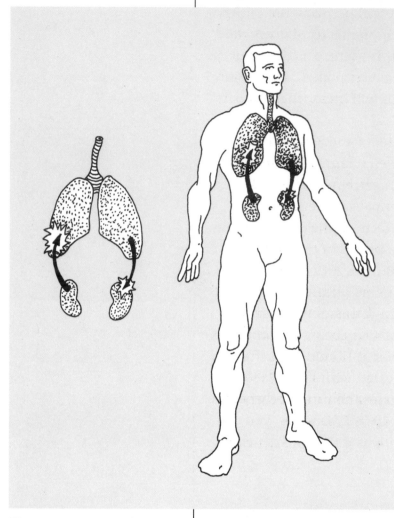

*Figure 14.* Lung-Kidney Relationship

As the Master of the Yinqiao Mai, KI 6 (Zhaohai) controls the distribution of yin energy to the upper part of the body, including the eyes. It ends at BL 1 (Jingming). KI 6 (Zhaohai) is useful for heat arising out of yin xu and fatigue. Gynecologically, it can be used to treat early period, menopause, premature graying, hot flashes, personality disturbances, chronic illness, and dry eyes, all signs of Kidney yin and essence deficiency. This point is used mainly for women.

Lung 7 (Lieque) is coupled with Kidney 6 (Zhaohai). The Lungs send their energy down and the Kidney grasps that qi and propels it upward *(see Figure 14)*. The image of the two channels together is similar to a wheel that puts stagnation in motion.

# 7. SI 3 (Houxi)

SI 3 (Houxi) is the shu (stream) point, the wood point, and the tonification point of the Small Intestine meridian. It is clinically effective for joint, bone and neck, and muscle and tendon problems. These symptoms frequently accompany essence deficiency diseases like menopause and infertility.

In Japanese acupuncture, SI 3 (Houxi) is considered a point that indicates the health of the pituitary gland.[1] Though it is somewhat awkward to palpate, a positive response can be elicited at the point. Houxi is an effective point for gynecological problems connected to the pituitary gland, the master gland of the body, which is responsible for hormonal regulation. Women with a tender SI 3 (Houxi) often have gynecological problems diagnosed as Kidney yang xu or stagnant blood arising from the use of birth control pills, which alter the hormonal environment of the user and cause Liver qi and blood stagnation.[2]

Small Intestine 3 (Houxi) is the Master point of the Du channel. As the Master point that governs all the yang channels, it aids in regulating the yang energy that arises upward via the Du channel. Thus, it affects the flow of energy from the Kidney through the spine, neck, head, and face. It increases the yang of the whole body.

## 8. BL 62 ( Shenmai)

Shenmai is the Master point of the Yangqiao Mai. It is responsible for absorbing excess yang energy in the upper part of the body all the way to the eyes, thus holding it down. Excess energy in the upper part of the body in the form of headache, personality disturbances, insomnia, and hot flashes that may accompany menopause can be treated with BL 62 (Shenmai). Governing Vessel energy manipulated by using SI 3 (Houxi), lifts energy from the lower part of the body. This is the image of how these two points work together.

1. Matsumoto K: Workshop on palpation. Southwest Acupuncture College, Santa Fe, N.M., July, 1988.

2. Flaws B: The pill and stagnant blood: the side-effects of oral contraceptives according to traditional Chinese medicine. *J Chi Med,* 1990; 32: 19–21.

Although BL 62 (Shenmai) is coupled with SI 3 (Houxi), it can be used gynecologically with KI 6. This is an effective combination for the hot flashes associated with menopause, particularly if the patient also has signs and symptoms of underlying Kidney deficiency. The combination of these points regulates the yin and yang energy of the heel that travels to the head; these points together absorb excess energy in that area. The treatment consists of tonifying KI 6 (Zhaohai), dispersing BL 62 (Shenmai), and also dispersing BL 1 (Jingming).

In summary, we see that the Confluent points possess energetics that are widely applicable to the treatment of gynecological problems as well as other conditions. They can be needled singularly, in combination with their coupled Confluent point, or used as the skeletal basis of treatment. The palpation and needling of the Eight Confluent points can be found in *Table 28* (see Chapter Eleven).

**Case 9.** The treatment of menopause with the Eight Curious Vessels

The patient was a forty-seven-year-old-female whose major complaint was of menopausal symptoms that had begun two weeks previously. The signs and symptoms included hot flashes, dull hot abdominal pain, hip pain, feelings of craziness and disorientation, night sweats, extreme thirst, occipital headaches, itchy skin, depression and sadness, fatigue, worry, heavy limbs, poor sleep, facial breakouts, lots of gas, neck and back pain, canker sores, dream-disturbed sleep, and constipation. She had been taking estrogen therapy for those two weeks, but had decided to discontinue it because the hormones had not worked and because of a history of fibrocystic tumors in both herself and her family.

The tongue was pale, swollen, and short with a red tip and sides, a thick, yellow, greasy coat, and a central crack. She had thick, coarse, gray hair. Her lips were purple; the face dry and wrinkled. Her body was short and stocky and she wore tight jewelry and tight clothing. The pulse was weak, thready, and rapid on the left and slippery on the right.

From age and a lifestyle that included a lot of stress, and from poor nutrition and alcohol, the qi of the Kidney was weak. The patient manifested signs and symptoms of Kidney qi xu, that is both yin and yang deficiency, and that produced symptoms of hot and cold blood with blood deficiency. This further led to symptoms of Heart and Spleen blood deficiency.

The diagnosis was depletion of Kidney essence, Liver blood and yin deficiency, Liver qi stagnation, Heart and Spleen qi and blood xu. The etiology and pathogenesis of her case was from the natural decline of Kidney qi exacerbated by stress, diet, lifestyle factors, alcohol, and her underlying constitution. The treatment plan was to tonify the Kidney essence and to tonify the qi and the blood.

*continued*

To get a sense of the whole person, as well as the complexity of the case, I have provided the answers to the Ten Questions and observations that represent pathological data.

- neck tension
- depression
- facial breakouts
- shoulders frequently hurt
- pain at the vertex
- overreacts
- on synthyroid for multiple goiters from forty years of age
- two fibrocystic tumors in left breast
- agitated, weepy
- history of erratic period, once spotted for two months

- darkness under the eyes
- headaches at Taiyang
- pain in the inguinal region
- ovarian cyst removed at twenty-five years of age
- sciatic pain
- lower lumbar/sacral pain at the iliac crest
- craves salads, vegetables
- craziness, "spaciness," disorientation
- feeling of organs sinking
- eats lot of frozen yogurt
- periodically eats spoiled food

Acupuncture was administered for a period of ten weeks, two times a week. The treatment improved the hip, eliminated the headaches and the abdominal pain, cooled the skin, calmed the spirit, reduced the hot flashes and the insomnia, and improved morale. There had been an adverse reaction to herbs in the past with another practitioner and the patient was hesitant to try herbs again. However, herbs were introduced into therapy in the third week and they further diminished the hot flashes. At this point a correlation could always be made between the hot flashes and stress.

The patient was very compliant in receiving treatments on a regular basis and only took the herbs because of her trust in the practitioner. She was reluctant to change her lifestyle habits of late nights, alcohol, tight clothing, and did not take measures to reduce stress. As of the last follow-up, ten months after treatment stopped, the patient relied only upon one herbal tablet per day to control the hot flashes. Her nipples changed from postpregnancy brown to the color of a young girl's. Mental symptoms subsided after six treatments. The balance of the treatments (fourteen) improved tongue color to a light red, reduced its flabbiness, cleared the thick, yellow greasy coat to a thin white, and eliminated all symptoms, reducing the hot flashes from five times an hour to once a day.

Advice to the patient centered around the following:

1. Reducing stress, anxiety, and worry

2. Maintaining bone strengthening exercises

3. Eating balanced, nutritious meals; reducing overconsumption of raw cold food, salads, frozen yogurt, and spoiled foods

4. Reduction/elimination of alcohol and late-night entertainment

5. Receiving acupuncture supplemented with auricular acupuncture, and taking herbs.

Specifically, I put her on a course of Fem-Estro, Cal-Apatite, and Recovery of Youth Tablets (see discussion of these products in Chapter Eighteen on menopause). Prior to selecting these, she had had poor results with Liu Wei Di Huang Wan and Placenta Restorative Tablets. The first one produced lots of gas (probably due to the yin nature of the rehmannia root and her preexisting Spleen qi xu). The second one made her itchy, which was perhaps an allergic reaction to the human placenta (another person's protein).

*continued*

Treatment with the Eight Curious Vessels, although not exclusive, was a fundamental part of the treatment strategy. Throughout the course of treatment all of the Confluent points of the Eight Curious Vessels were used, based on the signs, symptoms, and the pattern of relationships she had on the day of treatment. A few of these points were always part of her treatment. The energetics of these points were explained in this chapter.

The two points at the core of her treatment were KI 6 (Zhaohai) and BL 62 (Shenmai). Table 28 (see Chapter Eleven) outlines the unique locations and needle techniques for each point. The actions of these points are as follows.

KI 6 is the primary point for yin deficiency anywhere in the body. Part of the reason is that KI 6 is also the Master point of the Yinqiao Mai. In this role, KI 6 regulates the energy of the yin vessels of the heel. The energy of this vessel, which travels to the upper part of the body and brings yin energy with it, ends at BL 1 (Jingming). We want this effect in the case of menopause involving Kidney yin deficiency. The point is tonified.

BL 62 (Shenmai), is the Master of the Yangqiao Mai. This meridian regulates the energy of the yang meridians of the heel. It brings yang energy from the head and upper part of the body downward. The point is helpful in menopause when the yang of the body is rising. BL 62 is dispersed.

In combination, these two points effectively combat yin/yang disharmony, a characteristic of menopause.

# A SYNOPSIS OF BLOODLETTING TECHNIQUES

## General Principles

Included in the repertoire of the Nine Ancient needles expounded upon in the *Lingshu* was the use of the three-edge needle *(Figure 15).* The modern three-edge needle is derived from this early type. It is obvious from inspecting this needle that the tip does not have the usual pine needle configuration of filiform needles. Rather, it has a triangular head designed to make a larger hole in the skin for bloodletting. Because these needles are hard to locate or are of such a quality that their tips are jagged and can actually damage tissue, practitioners frequently substitute medical lancets for the same purpose. Ordinary acupuncture needles can also be used and in this case, a large gauge needle such as a #28 or #30 should be selected.

The three-edge needle was produced to treat clinical conditions through the following three therapeutic aims:

1. To promote the smooth flow of qi and blood in the meridians or tissues, so as to

The Bleeding Needle

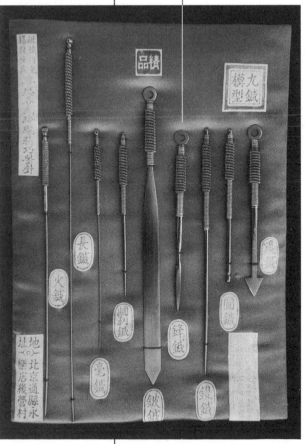

***Figure 15.*** The Nine Ancient Needles

clear the channels.

2. To dispel blood stasis and activate qi and blood by promoting its unobstructed flow, and

3. To drain heat-fire.

Clinical conditions that are manifestations of these disorders will be discussed later in this chapter.

The anatomical locations of most of the points that are bled are relatively shallow places such as superficial blood vessels.  Other commonly bled points include ear points, scalp points, and jing (well) points that are located close to the surface.  Jing (well) points in particular lend themselves to bleeding not only because of their location but also because of their inherent energy.

As the most distal points on a meridian, farthest away from the center of energy in the body, jing (well) points are sites where the energy of a meridian is like water filling a well.  The energy is just starting to appear and bubble.  From a Five Element point of view, the use of these points is particularly appropriate for the Spring season as well as the "Spring" of a disease, that is, the early, acute stages of a disorder.  At the nexus of the jing (well) points, the qualities of yin and yang are less differentiated and tend to merge, hence they are especially beneficial in effecting a rapid transformation of energy from yang to yin and yin to yang.  Thus these points are useful for balance, for expelling fullness in the organs, and for changing polarity.

In bleeding techniques, speed is essential in puncturing the point to reduce sustained contact with free nerve endings.  The depth of insertion for these points is very shallow ranging between .05-.1 cun.

The most common form of manipulation of the bloodletting needle is the spot pricking or collateral pricking technique (collaterals referring to the meridians and vessels).  Most points, such as jing (well) points, are punctured in this manner.  Prior to inserting the needle, the point should be massaged or squeezed to cause slight venous pooling so that when the needle is inserted, blood will be released. After the skin is pricked and a small puncture is made so that blood is extracted, a clean cotton ball should be applied to the site and pressed firmly to absorb the droplets and stop the bleeding. An adhesive bandage should also be put over the puncture site to prevent any infection until the puncture has healed.

A second technique involves making tiny pinprick motions to the affected area until blood is released. This method is referred to as clumping or area pricking. The technique is suitable for reddened skin tissue, bruising and extravasation, or other overt signs of blood stagnation. After the punctures have been made, the epidermis should be squeezed to obtain more blood. Following the escape of the blood, it should be absorbed with a sterile piece of cotton gauze and then covered with an adhesive bandage or antiseptic solution, again to prevent infection.

Next, bloodletting can be facilitated by pinching the skin with the nondominant hand and pricking the affected area with a three-edge needle to induce bleeding. Other devices such as the Plum Blossom (Seven Star or cutaneous needle), a regular filiform needle, or the shoni-shin needle can be employed to stimulate a large area so that superficial bleeding occurs.

All contraindications for needling apply in bloodletting. If the patient has generalized weakness, anemia, a hypotensive condition, hemorrhagic disease, or is pregnant or recently delivered, bloodletting should not be used. The course of treatment varies from one treatment or until the condition is rectified. Treat once per day or on alternate days. If the patient bleeds a lot, treat one to two times per week.

A survey of the indications of the acupuncture points of the body reveals that numerous points lend themselves to bleeding, and indeed in the clinical conditions listed in *Table 29*, bleeding is the method of choice to bring about the desired therapeutic result.

*Table 29.* The Bleeding Needle: Points to Needle for Specific Clinical Conditions

| POINTS | CONDITIONS |
|---|---|
| LU 11 | Sore throat of the excess type, i.e., exogenous invasion, tonsillitis, stuffiness and pain in chest, asthmatic breathing, stomachache, frontal shoulder pain |
| LI 1 | Toothache, sore throat, nasal obstruction, tinnitus, frontal headache, stomachache, shoulder pain |
| HT 9 | Febrile diseases, stuffiness and pain in the chest, palpitations, angina pectoris, insomnia, headache, tinnitus, shoulder pain, back pain |
| SI 1 | Febrile diseases |
| BL 2 | Wind-heat in the eyes, acute conjunctivitis |
| BL 40 | Back pain, acute lumbar sprain, multiple furuncles and swelling, sunstroke, leg pain |
| PC 3 | Febrile disease, acute vomiting |
| PC 9 | Coma, unconsciousness, stuffiness and pain in chest, palpitations, angina, insomnia, stomach problems, pain in Liver region |
| TE 1 | Tinnitus, migraine, sore throat, shoulder pain, back pain, pain in the chest and hypochondriac region, hepatic distending pain |
| GV 4 | Lumbago |
| GV 14 and its Huatoujiaji's* | Lung heat (excess) |
| GV 26 | Lumbago |
| **EXTRA POINTS:** | |
| Taiyang | Acute conjunctivitis, hypertension |
| Erjian (ear apex) | Acute conjunctivitis, spasms, high fever caused by toxicity, wind, heat, Liver yang rising |
| Jinjin and Yuyue (veins under tongue) | Pernicious vomiting, aphasia |
| Shixuan (tips of fingers) | Coma, epilepsy, infantile convulsion, sunstroke |
| Sifeng (midpoint of interphalangeal joints of all fingers except thumb) | Digestive disorders in children (prick when purple; white fluid may come out) |
| Baxie (junction of margin of webs of fingers) | Spasm and contracture of the fingers (pathologic fluid may come out) |
| Local | Varicose veins, phlebitis |
| Jing (well) points | Numbness, stroke |
| **COMBINATIONS:** | |
| LI 4, LI 11 | Numbness |
| ST 36, GV 26, PC 3, BL 40, PC 6, Jing (well) points | Hypertension |
| BL 40, LU 5, ST 44, PC 3 | Sunstroke, acute gastroenteritis |

*\*The Huatoujiaji points mentioned here are a group of points on both sides of the spinal column at the lateral borders of each spinous process from the first thoracic vertebra to the fifth lumbar vertebra. For more information, see* Essentials of Chinese Acupuncture, *Beijing College of Traditional Chinese Medicine, Foreign Language Press, compiled by Beijing, PRC, 1980, pp 291–292.*

*Table 29* correlates common clinical conditions with the bleeding needle. However, the indications are by no means exhaustive. Inflammation, with its characteristic signs of redness, swelling, and pain is well-treated through this method. For example, for a swollen ankle, a Plum Blossom needle is used. This treatment is generally quite painful when administered but is also unsurpassed in activating the flow of qi and blood to the affected area.  The prognosis is greatly enhanced and the resolution is accelerated by this technique.  Red, swollen, painful arthritis, neurodermatitis, allergic dermatitis, rhinitis, headache, erysipelas, lymphatitis, and hemorrhoids can also be treated in this way.

# The Treatment of Blood Stasis with Bleeding Techniques

We have seen that bleeding techniques are invaluable in the treatment of blood stasis because of their ability to promote the free flow of qi and blood, to disperse blood stasis, and to eliminate heat.  A rather serious manifestation of blood stasis and accumulation at the base of the occiput can occur in cases of high blood pressure as an early sign of stroke.  It resembles a large bruise or birth mark and ranges in color from red to dark purple.

Anatomically, the occiput is predisposed to energetic blockages because it is a physical protuberance.  Qi stagnation in the form of neck tension, subluxated vertebrae, and arthritic bone deformities are common manifestations of this predisposition.  When blood stagnation develops in this area, it is an unfavorable condition that needs to be treated immediately with the modality of choice, bloodletting.

As a prestroke manifestation, the patient generally has a history of hypertension or minimally labile blood pressure, that is, the person's blood pressure changes in response to environmental stimuli.  Because it appears at the base of the skull, usually in the GB 20 (Fengchi) area, patients are generally not aware of the presence of the extravasated blood because they cannot see it.  Other signs and symptoms will prompt the skilled practitioner to examine this area.  These symptoms include severe emotional distress, an odd sensation in the tongue, and facial numbness on the side where the ecchymosis is present. In addition, the patient will probably have a deviated tongue, an early sign of windstroke. If the patient mentions the tongue and facial sensations, the practitioner should immediately inspect the neck and treat it if the blood stasis is present.

Blood stasis, a physical blockage, represents a potential embolism and/or a blockage that can lead to the creation of internal wind, which can be a precipitating factor in the development of stroke. The stasis must be dispelled immediately to avert such a dangerous situation. If the patient is simultaneously noting the tongue and facial discomfort, it indicates that the Heart is involved and that there is a lack of blood flow to the face. I know of no sources that state, "If the tongue feels 'weird,' there is Heart involvement." However, the tongue as the sprout of the Heart suggests some connection, and my clinical experience verifies this.

Under these conditions it is imperative to disperse the blood stasis. We can do this with any number of tools that can produce bloodletting, such as the Plum Blossom needle, the tri-edge needle, a filiform needle, or shoni-shin needle. How to use each of these instruments is summarized in *Table 30*.

Only draw a small amount of blood with these techniques; the droplets may actually be very small, but they should be present and make the breakup and invigoration of qi and blood obvious. Although this is a highly specific treatment for a unique clinical condition and is very beneficial for the patient, the practitioner should not risk her or his own health by exposure to blood-borne pathogens. Follow OSHA (Occupation, Safety, and Health Administration) guidelines. As in all cases of pricking, clean needle technique must be employed: needles must be sterile, and it is highly advisable for the practitioner to wear a double pair of gloves as well as a facial mask. Goggles are also recommended to protect the practitioner from the aerosolized blood that can be generated by a vigorous bloodletting style.

*Table 30.* Bloodletting Techniques for Blood Stasis Patterns in the Occipital Area

| INSTRUMENT | METHOD |
|---|---|
| Plum Blossom needle | Quickly and vigorously tap the skin of the affected area so that a slight amount of blood is released. Carefully absorb the blood with a sterile piece of gauze and dispose of it properly. Re-usable or disposable Plum Blossom needles may be used. Sterilize or dispose of properly. |
| Bleeding needle | With a specialized bleeding needle (tri-edge needle) repeatedly pierce the affected area. If this needle or a medical lancet is used, more blood will be extracted because of the size of the needle tip. Use the same quick and vigorous insertion technique, but pierce less frequently over the same skin area if you want less bleeding. |
| Filiform needle | Quickly and vigorously pierce the affected area. Repeatedly release small droplets of blood as with the Plum Blossom and tri-edge needle techniques. Use a #28 or #30 gauge needle. Some patients tolerate the repeated insertion of this needle better than the piercing done by the Plum Blossom needle, which can be aggravating because of the number of needles in its head. It is also less painful than a lancet or a tri-edge needle because of its smaller tip. This is my preferred method of bloodletting. |
| Shoni-shin needle | This small plastic pediatric needle can also be substituted for any of the previous techniques. The clinical utility of this needle, apart from its effectiveness, is that it is plastic and disposable, whereas the reusable Plum Blossom needle needs to be sterilized before reuse. Also, the patients can keep the needle and treat themselves. (Note: Before disposal of the shoni-shin needle, please sterilize.) |

Apart from cases of hypertension, other patients with labile blood pressure may also develop blood stasis in situations of emotional distress. Usually, they are aware of something going on in the occipital area because the skin becomes unbearably itchy there. Inspection by the practitioner reveals the characteristic blood stagnation mark. Although any of the above methods can be used to invigorate the smooth flow of qi and blood and thus disperse the blood stagnation, the shoni-shin needle is the most practical because the patient can keep the needle for self-treatment. In addition, the opposite end of this needle has a scraping edge that can also be used by the patient to move the qi and blood and relieve itchiness without piercing the skin, similar to the modality of gwa sha.

*Cases 10* and *11* illustrate the clinical use of blood-letting techniques.

| **Case 10.** Blood stasis patterns in the occipital region

The patient was a seventy-four-year-old female with many serious health problems. She sought acupuncture treatment primarily for the effects of knee surgery and a car accident. She had shooting pains in her thighs and left big toe. Other health problems included high blood pressure, arthritis, a personal history of heart attack, and extreme emotional agitation from family problems. There were many other complaints that unfolded weekly from this friendly and talkative patient. At the time of the initial intake, I noticed that the tongue was grossly enlarged and deviated. Regardless of how the patient was doing from week to week, this fact always concerned me.

The patient was inconsistent in taking her high blood pressure medication because of its cost. I could not convince her of the danger of this practice and even had a medical doctor explain the seriousness of not taking her medication regularly, but to no avail.

The patient received acupuncture treatments twice a week and responded favorably. Within five months, many of her problems were resolved as well as most symptoms related to the major complaint. However, there were still symptoms that I was particularly concerned about. These included dizziness, cold sweats, a weak quivery voice, armpit pain, numbness of the left arm, fatigue, and insomnia. In addition, the patient reported that her tongue felt swollen and that it burned. She could feel her heart on the left side, her left arm hurt, she was tired, and had "heartburn." Her left eye was hard to close and felt heavy. She also had occasional flashes in her head and her blood pressure remained consistently high. I insisted that she see her heart specialist immediately, but she refused because of the cost of tests, time constraints, and a feeling of lack of rapport and trust with the specialists.

Acupuncture treatment temporarily brought her blood pressure down and the head flashes stopped. The patient finally saw her cardiologist after I made an appointment for her. The blood pressure continued to stay elevated, she felt pressure on the left side of the head, her lips felt numb, and her eyes were blurry. These symptoms suggested an imminent heart attack or stroke. At this point, I inspected the base of the skull and saw the characteristic blood stasis hematoma.

I immediately explained the Plum Blossom bloodletting technique to the patient and began to treat the affected area. Within seconds the patient reported that the "weird" feeling in her tongue was diminishing. After a few minutes of therapy the facial numbness and heaviness were gone. The effects of this treatment lasted for about three weeks.

One month later the patient reported many serious symptoms: four nights of insomnia due to palpitations, shortness of breath made worse by laying down, feeling her heart pound in her ears, head distention, generalized stiffness on the left side, her mouth feeling funny, a feeling of a "dead" spot on the right side of her face, "heartburn," sleeping in the day, swollen feet, numbness of the arms and legs, feeling like she weighed "500 pounds," and a bitter taste in the mouth. She had a deep red tongue and a fast pulse. Also, her high blood pressure, for which she was not taking her medication, continued.

Treatment with the Plum Blossom needle helped diminish the numbness, heaviness, and weird feelings, however, the patient was admonished to seek Western medical help. Two weeks later she admitted herself to the emergency room as she finally recognized the seriousness of her problem. She explained to the doctor that an acupuncturist had been treating her for prestroke symptoms and he told her that the bloodletting treatment she received had probably prevented her from having a stroke. The easy sweat and tiredness with lack of exertion continued and further medical tests revealed low levels of oxygen in the blood.

Shortly thereafter the patient's insurance company would no longer pay for her acupuncture treatment since the major complaint of trauma-related injuries was resolved. Even though I offered her unlimited free treatments, the patient had already run up bills that the insurance company would not pay when the emphasis in treatment changed, and her pride would not allow her to accept free treatment.

I cautioned her to take her medications and to see her cardiologist. I told her as well to call if she needed any further treatment that she thought I could offer her.

**Case 11.** Additional case of blood stasis patterns in the occipital region

The patient was a thirty-five-year-old female with an acute complaint of unbearable scalp itchiness. She was applying a corticosteroid cream, which was recommended by a dermatologist. Also, she was using a Chinese liniment prescribed by a private practitioner. Neither solution was working.

One day, in passing, she mentioned to me that these modalities were not helping and that she was desperate. At the same time, she was experiencing a series of family tragedies. In characteristic fashion, she was taking on and internalizing all these problems, and she told me that she had not given herself the time to cry yet. She had tightness in the chest and throat, extreme grief, anger, and heightened irritability. Inspection of the patient confirmed that she had a tendency to hold things in. Her complexion was greenish-black with an underlying sallowness to it. Her blood pressure was generally low, but could become situationally labile.

Because I was going to see what I could do on an emergency basis, I used what I had gained from observation as well as minimal but focused questioning. When I asked to see where the itchiness was, the patient pointed to the base of the occiput in the GV 15-16, GB 20 area. I could clearly see the characteristic blood stasis pattern.

I began repeatedly piercing the ecchymosis while the patient sat with her head bent forward onto a desk. Dark red-black blood began to emerge, and within one minute the patient reported that the unbearable itchiness that had plagued her for weeks was gone. To disperse the stasis I advised her to scratch the affected area with the comb-like edge of the shoni-shin needle if the itchiness recurred. I also told her to disperse the stasis and to apply Zheng Gu Shui to the affected area if the needle did not help to further invigorate the blood. Shortly after the treatment, the grief from her suppressed emotions began to be released and the problem was totally resolved.

# Common Uses of the Plum Blossom Needle

Apart from conditions where bloodletting is desired, the Plum Blossom needle as a vehicle for facilitating the free flow of qi and blood can also be used. This section addresses some difficult-to-treat conditions where the Plum Blossom needle can be used effectively. These conditions include myopia and other eye problems, baldness, varicose veins, the common cold, constipation, migraines, and acute conjunctivitis. *Table 31* outlines the clinical condition and the corresponding method of treatment to use with the Plum Blossom needle and *Case 12* describes an effective application of this technique. Do not apply to the face, ulcerations, or to weak patients.

*Table 31.* The Treatment of Common Clinical Conditions with the Plum Blossom Needle

| CONDITION | TREATMENT |
|---|---|
| Eye problems, such as myopia, lacrimation, and atrophy of the optic nerve | Plum Blossom LI 14 (Binao), GB 37 (Guangming), Taiyang, and an extra point between the eyebrow and the eyeball, GB 20 (Fengchi) due to its relationship to the visual cortex in the occipital lobe, GV 14 (Dazhui), PC 6 (Neiguan) to regulate the qi and blood of the entire body. Also, as Master of the Yinwei Mai brings energy to the eyes. ST 1 (Chengqi), and GB 1 (Tonziliao). Supplement with the following auricular points for good effect: Eye 1, 2, 3, occiput, shenmen, LR, ST, SP, KI. |
| Baldness (especially an acute onset) | Tap heavily over the affected area, then apply fresh ginger juice. |
| Varicose veins* | Tap very lightly on the protruding veins; do not try to elicit blood. Use a zigzag motion over the veins. |
| Common cold | Tap along the medial Bladder lines, as well as along both sides of the nose. |
| Constipation | Administer on the lower abdomen and on the back in the lumbar-sacral region. |
| Migraine | Tap on the nape of the neck on the affected side, on PC 6 (Neiguan), TE 5 (Waiguan), and in the sacral region. |
| Acute conjunctivitis | Tap in the area of the cervical vertebrae (C1–4), around the eyes, on GB 20 (Fengchi), Taiyang, and LI 4 (Hegu). |

*\* The Chinese doctors I studied with differentiate varicose veins as a Kidney, not a Spleen problem, since it occurs in the lower jiao and is generally accompanied by edema. Also, older people tend to develop it.*

**Case 12.** The application of the Plum Blossom needle in the treatment of hair loss

The patient was a forty-eight-year-old woman whose major complaint was hair loss. At the time she came to seek Chinese medical treatment the problem had been going on for six years. Since onset she lost about half of her hair, most of it from the right side. The problem had become more pronounced within the last year.

Her hair was coming out by the roots. Its texture was dry and the color was fading. The patient's scalp felt tight around the crown area and the tightness was worsened by stress. She felt pinpricking pain on the right side of her scalp and at the base of her skull, so much so that the pain woke her up at night. She also felt cold on that side of her head. Her hair was thin, particularly around the Gall Bladder and other yang channels of the head. The patient presented with several other major complaints, many health problems, and subpathologies.

In treating this chronic problem, it was important that the patient's major complaint not be isolated from the context of who she was, that is, from all of her health problems. However, without enumerating them all, the patient's root diagnosis was blood deficiency leading to blood stagnation.

The pattern of hair loss is clearly one of deficiency, specifically of the blood. The hair is the extension of the blood and the head hair belongs to the Kidney. All of her signs and symptoms including weak left superficial pulses and the pale, thin, dry tongue suggested a blood deficiency.

There was some blood stagnation in the head from the deficiency and this created the tight feeling over the crown area and the pinpricking sensation. The treatment principle was directed at tonifying the blood, dispersing blood stagnation, and tonifying the qi of the Kidney. Many treatment modalities were selected for the patient, including Plum Blossom needling, moxa, acupuncture, herbal therapy, nutritional counseling, and exercise advice.

To address the major complaint, the Plum Blossom needle was selected as the tool of choice for the affected area followed by an application of fresh ginger juice. Even though the hair loss was a long-term problem, this strategy had the combined effect of dispersing stagnation as well as increasing circulation to the affected area. Moxibustion was administered in the form of the moxa box on the abdomen to tonify the internal deficiency that had manifested as blood deficiency and internal cold. Acupuncture was selected to adjust the qi and blood. Herbs were chosen to build as well as move blood. Dietary counseling was critical to compensate for a history of poor eating habits along with a vegetarian diet that together had further weakened the body's capacity to produce blood and anchor the hair, so to speak. Exercise regimes were discussed to strengthen the qi and blood as well as move the stagnation.

The patient received treatment in the office three times a month for three months and then came back for a final treatment and consultation two months later. The patient took herbs, tried to eat better, and administered the Plum Blossom technique on herself. After the first treatment, which included the Plum Blossom technique to the GV 20 (Baihui) and GB 20 (Fengchi) areas, the scalp tightness was reduced and her energy level was higher. Three weeks later she only experienced one night of pricking scalp pain and no scalp tightness, even though she had been extremely stressed. By her tenth and final treatment the hair loss had stopped, the pricking pain had abated, and there was almost no head tension. When head tension did develop the patient could always correlate it with stress that she was not managing. These results were maintained for three years without further treatment.

In my opinion, the success of this treatment, not only with regard to the major complaint but also as to many of the patient's other serious health problems, was based on the recognition of the common denominator of all of her health problems. Excellent patient compliance and herbal therapy enhanced the effects. This is an interesting case of a complex blood deficiency problem manifesting as hair loss that was well treated through augmenting the simple yet appropriate tool of the Plum Blossom needle.

# Gwa Sha:  Scraping Evil Wetness

Supplementing the tapping and bleeding techniques designed to treat the manifestations of blood stasis is another modality, that of *gwa sha*, a scraping mechanism. Although it is not technically a bleeding technique, its effects are so similar that I have included it here.

Gwa sha, translated as "scraping evil wetness" or "scraping sand," can be used in two manifestations of evil wetness accumulating in the body. There can be either stagnant blood or dampness in the body as secondary pathological products, or both. In the case of blood stagnation from an internal or miscellaneous origin from qi deficiency, retardation in the flow of qi and blood, trauma or injury, this scraping technique helps to activate the abnormal or obstructed flow of qi and blood in the joints and muscles.

As far as dampness is concerned, gwa sha is helpful for obstruction caused by internal qi deficiency, not by an external invasion of wind, cold, damp, or heat into the body. It is important to note that if a rheumatic bi syndrome is treated with this technique, it is likely to recur since it was inappropriate for gwa sha.

The scraping motion of gwa sha is executed with a firm-edged tool such as a pediatric scraping needle, the comb-like edge of the shoni-shin needle or any other similar device. I prefer to use the firm edge of a Chinese soup spoon; it is not only aesthetic and comfortable in the hand but does the job well. Using a brisk, short, flicking action, the chosen apparatus is applied over the affected area in a simultaneous top-to-bottom and medial-to-lateral direction. This vigorous, superficial massage technique improves the circulation of qi and blood to the affected area. Points of the body that are commonly treated with gwa sha include the neck, joints, legs, abdomen, back, and musculoskeletal regions. Because we are trying to move stagnation, this vigorous technique may result in bruising, tenderness, tiredness, or invigoration, and the patient should be informed of these possible side effects.

For added result, gwa sha can be used in combination with appropriate acupuncture points. Liniments can also be used to move qi and blood and to clear the channels. Some of the most effective solutions are Zheng Gu Shui, Possum On, Woodlock Oil, Regal Oil, and Tieh Ta Yao Gin. Apply an ample amount of the selected oil to the affected area and then administer the gwa sha technique. Apply less vigorously to patients with delicate skin or to those who bruise easily. Scrape the affected area once with each stroke, making your way from top to bottom. Repeat this procedure three to five times depending upon the reaction. The area should become visibly red, but do not break the skin or induce bleeding.

Zheng Gu Shui and Tieh Ta Yao Gin have the added benefit of resolving blood stasis that may have been the condition treated in the first place. They can dispel any blood stasis in the form of bruising that may have resulted from the technique. Cupping over the area that was treated with gwa sha is another common combined Chinese modality. Lubricating liniments such as Regal Oil, Possum On, Woodlock Oil, and Wan Hua can be applied to the skin prior to the gwa sha and the cupping. When the cups are removed, the blood dispersing liniments can be reapplied to the area just treated to continue to move the stasis and resolve any ecchymosis.

Never do gwa sha over an open wound, sore, scar, skin eruption, or on contagious skin rashes. The spoon must be sterilized for each new patient. If other scraping instruments are used, they, too, should be sterilized or, if they are disposable, disposed of properly as with the shoni-shin needle.

Treating these unique patterns of blood stasis with the techniques described here is not just a symptomatic treatment of the disorder. Rather, it is a root approach that invigorates stagnant qi and blood, and thus addresses the underlying etiology. The way patients handle their emotions should be pointed out to them so they can recognize how they are expressing their feelings through their bodies. In cases of blood pressure problems, patients should use Western medical techniques in addition to Oriental methods.

# CHAPTER 14

# PERICARDIUM 6
## Gate to Internal Well-being

As the "Inner Gate,"[1] Pericardium 6 (Neiguan) ranks as one of the most important points for evaluating the internal state of the organism, whether that condition is designated as physical or psychological. Any stagnation or deficiency in the body, but particularly qi stagnation, can be both measured and treated through palpation that evokes objective reactions from the patient or subjective impressions in the practitioner. Impressions include tissue tension, tendon hardness, point mushiness, or tight or loose spacing of the tendons. Stagnation is constantly cited as the root cause of much illness, so the clinical utility of assessing stagnation becomes apparent. The ease of palpating this point makes it possible for patients to monitor their own health and empowers them to address their life situations so they can restore their own internal harmony.

In 1987, during a lecture on the Eight Curious Vessels, the esteemed Nguyen Van Nghi, M.D., reviewed a case that illustrated the application of PC 6 (Neiguan). He told us that on his flight from Paris to the United States, a passenger had become ill and unconscious. The flight attendant requested medical help to deal with the emergency. Dr. Van Nghi, both a medical

---

1. Maciocia G: *The Foundations of Chinese Medicine.* Churchill Livingston, London, 1989; p 435.

doctor and acupuncturist (as one must be to practice acupuncture in France), came to the assistance of the patient. Firmly, he reached for the wrist area of the patient where PC 6 (Neiguan) is located and the patient was revived.

When Dr. Van Nghi told this story, hands immediately went up in the classroom. Was the point needled or pressed? Was the treatment administered bilaterally or unilaterally? Were any other points used? Dr. Van Nghi, steeped in wisdom and experience, knew this would be the reaction; after all, practitioners want clinical information. With characteristic effusiveness he quickly brushed these questions aside to make his point: *When the specific nature, the distinct energetics, and the functions of each point in the body are truly understood, the number of points, the needling or pressing of the point unilaterally or bilaterally, and many other parameters of treatment become meaningless.*

This simple yet dramatic case illustrates concepts that are part of a general principle of treatment in Chinese medicine. Less is sometimes better and treating the root may be more productive than becoming seduced by the myriad symptoms of patients' complaints. To respond as he did to the immediacy and root of the problem demanded a clarity of thought, a precision of diagnosis, that comes from an intimate knowledge of point energetics. What these points do, and the ability to arrive at *the* point for each condition can only come from a knowledge of the internal pathways of the meridians and a classical comprehension of point energetics.

## Energetics of PC 6 (Neiguan)

This understanding of precise point function can elevate many rarely used points to greater clinical status. These points, because of their intersections and pathways, are important vortices of energy. PC 6 (Neiguan) certainly has always enjoyed high regard in terms of point functions because of its simultaneous capacity as a Luo point and a Confluent point of the Yinwei Mai. However, it has considerably more, perhaps less well-known (but not less significant), clinical energetics.

Before preceding with the palpation and treatment schematic of the point, I will discuss the multiple functions of PC 6 (Neiguan). The highlights of the information outlined here have been summarized in *Table 32* for added convenience in clinical usage.

*Table 32.* Summary of the Energetic Functions of PC 6 (Neiguan)

| | |
|---|---|
| A. | As Luo (Connecting) Point |
| | • Assists in communication between and treatment of the three jiaos |
| | • Measures how emotions are impinging on physiological function |
| | • Drains perverse energy (i.e., qi stagnation, blood stagnation and depressive Liver fire, from the upper jiao) |
| | • Keeps qi and blood flowing in their proper pathways |
| B. | As Group Luo of the Three Arm Yin |
| | • Regulates the qi and blood of the Three Arm Yin (meridians) thereby moving stagnation and stopping pain |
| C. | As Confluent (Master) Point of the Yinwei Mai |
| | • Measures and/or produces yin defensive energy |
| D. | Jueyin Energetic Layer in the Six Divisions |
| | • Moves Liver qi stagnation |
| E. | Coupled with the San Jiao According to the Five Elements |
| | • Assesses immune function |
| F. | Pericardium-Uterus-Kidney Relationship |
| | • Functional impairment may lead to qi insufficiency in the lower jiao or |
| | • Depressed qi may transform into fire, causing the development of stagnant qi or blood |
| | • Influences Heart, Liver, and Kidney Function |
| G. | Coupled with the Chong Mai and Its Confluent Point in the Eight Extra Vessels System |
| | • Assists Spleen and Kidney function |
| H. | Meeting Place of All the Curious Vessels |
| | • Supplements the body with essential energy |
| | • Absorbs perverse pathogenic energy |

## A. PC 6 (Neiguan) as Luo Connecting Point

As I discussed in Chapter Six, Luo points can be used in two ways, either as transverse or longitudinal vessels. With a transverse Luo, a stimulus can be sent to the coupled organ-meridian complex, in this case the San Jiao (see the discussion of Five Element coupling for further connections of Neiguan with San Jiao).

Located in the upper heater, PC 6 assists in communicating between the three jiaos. It has a particularly good effect on upper burner disturbances such as chest pain, cardiac pain, hiccup, diaphragmatic disorders, mental illness, and insomnia. However, it is also clinically effective in middle jiao symptoms such as gastric pain, vomiting, nausea, and motion sickness. PC 6 calms and harmonizes the stomach by promoting the functional qi of the middle burner. Lower jiao disharmonies such as abdominal pain and diarrhea can also be treated through this point.

As a longitudinal Luo, PC 6 (Neiguan) sends a stimulus to its own organ-meridian complex. The Pericardium, as the envelope that protects the heart, shields the heart from aberrant emotions and can be used as a barometer to measure what effects the emotions have on physiological function.

In one classical usage, Luo points were used as channels to drain off or disperse excessive, stuck, perverse energy.[2] Neiguan, with its close association with the upper jiao (chest and heart in particular), can treat clinical manifestations such as breast distention, tumors, cysts, and cancer of the breast. Any or all of these can occur if pathological energy is not drained. These developments are part of the sequelae of qi stagnation, blood stagnation, and often times depressive Liver fire.

Stimulating PC 6 as a longitudinal Luo activates the internal pathway of the channel. The Pericardium channel, originating in the chest, passes through its related organ, the pericardium, through its Front Mu point, CV 17 (which is also the influential point that dominates the qi, spreading the qi like a mist to every part of the body). The longitudinal Luo descends through the diaphragm to the abdomen, regulating the qi, keeping energy flowing in its proper pathway, and

2. Unschuld P: *Medicine in China, A History of Ideas*. University of California Press, Berkeley, 1985; p 82.

preventing the qi and blood from being reckless or rebellious.

## B. Group Luo of the Three Arm Yin

In this capacity, Neiguan binds the Three Arm Yin (Lung, Heart, and Pericardium) together; it thereby assists the function of the Lung, Heart, and Pericardium. As a result, this point controls and regulates the qi and blood of the heart, opens the heart orifice, and calms the spirit, mind, and heart.  It broadens and expands the diaphragm, decongests the chest, and controls the chest above the stomach.  If stagnation is part of the disharmony of these organs, it can be well determined at this point.  Because stagnation in Chinese medicine translates into pain, the proper treatment of this point reduces or stops pain—not a small accomplishment for the many millions who suffer from chronic pain.

## C. Confluent (Master) of the Yinwei Mai

*Wei* means "connection," as I have pointed out.  As the Master (controlling) point of all the yin organ-meridian complexes (Lung, Heart, Pericardium, Liver, Spleen, and Kidney), Neiguan wraps them together.  For this reason alone it is an effective point.  Since an additional function of the Yinwei channel is to contribute to yin defensive energy (i.e., those yin essential substances such as *ye* fluids,[3] jing, marrow, and blood that constitute the material basis of health), this can be verified to a certain extent by palpating PC 6.  The point will also stimulate defensive energy into production through treatment.

## D. Jueyin Energetic Level in the Six Divisions

In the Six Division paradigm, PC 6 (Neiguan) is inextricably bound with the Liver complex.  This energetic, coupled with Luo point usage and its internal pathway,

---

3. *Jin-ye* are the yang and yin pure fluids of the body, respectively.

allows Neiguan to relieve stagnant Liver qi. In my opinion, PC 6 is the most clinically effective point for dredging stagnant Liver qi. It is probably a lack of appreciation of this energetic that makes Neiguan so undervalued as a point for adjusting Liver qi stagnation.

## E. Coupled in the Five Elements with the San Jiao

One of the functions of the San Jiao is to unite all three heaters so that it can produce and distribute the essential substances of qi, blood, body fluid, jing, shen, and marrow to the organism. For that reason it aids in immunity since these substances constitute the integrity and the building blocks of health. Assessing immune function then becomes an important energetic of this point.

## F. The Pericardium-Uterus-Kidney Relationship

Between the Pericardium (*xin bao*, the envelope that protects the heart) and the uterus (*Bao gong*, the envelope or palace of the child) there is a special internal pathway or vessel called the *Bao mai*. Another special vessel, the *Bao Luo*, connects the Kidney to the uterus, so the Pericardium has an intimate and complex connection with the uterus and Kidney *(see Figure 16)*. When qi stagnates or depresses in the chest, usually because of habitual emotional factors, there are two likely scenarios.

Insufficient qi may be transferred to the lower jiao (leading to Kidney qi deficiency) with resulting prob-

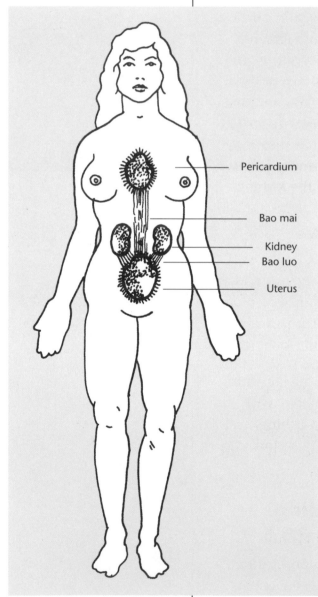

Pericardium

Bao mai

Kidney
Bao luo

Uterus

*Figure 16.* Pericardium-Uterus-Kidney Relationship

lems of amenorrhea, infertility, or other qi deficiency symptoms. Also, depressed qi may transform into fire. This causes heat to be conferred to the lower jiao with stagnant qi and blood manifestations developing such as clots, dysmenorrhea, or fibroid tumors. Thus, the use of PC 6 is a direct way of influencing Heart, Liver, and Kidney energy.

### G.  Coupled with the Chong Mai and SP 4 (Gongsun) in the Eight Extra Meridian System

Coupled to the Yinwei Mai, the Chong Mai has been described as virtually identical to the Kidney meridian, the only difference being that the Chong Mai is more superficial. Their Master points, SP 4 (Gongsun) and PC 6 (Neiguan) respectively, work closely and homeostatically together. The Spleen helps produce and distribute basic body materials via the San Jiao, and the Kidney provides the pilot light for those metabolic activities. Thus, the Spleen, Pericardium, and Kidney assist each other in basic body functions.

### H.  All the Eight Curious Vessels (Extra Meridians) connect here

This means that Neiguan is a very useful point for manipulating the energy of the Eight Curious Vessels. The action from PC 6 on the Extra Meridians falls into two major categories: supplementing the body with essential energy (yuan or original qi) or absorbing perverse pathogenic energy. Either of these actions can have important therapeutic results.

## Assessment of Clinical Findings Derived from Palpation of PC 6 (Neiguan)

After outlining the functions of PC 6 (Neiguan), it becomes apparent that it surely ranks as a remarkable point. Let me emphasize again that one of the key functions of PC 6 (Neiguan) is its ability to move Liver qi stagnation. As one anonymous observer said, "Give me Liver qi or give me death," a catchy phrase that restates the axiom, "The Six Stagnations are frequently the root of disease." Qi stagnation often arises from dysfunction of the Liver and can be the precursor to all other stagnations.

In Chinese medicine, stagnation, like many entities, has its gradations and nuances that define it. In establishing any diagnosis, sufficient signs and symptoms need to support each other, and stagnation is no exception. Its early manifestations are often subclinical, that is, below the threshold of overt perception or complaint. Regrettably, there is a tendency in Chinese medicine both in the United States, and perhaps even more in contemporary China, to ignore the importance of bodily palpation in evaluating the patient's condition.

The intent of this chapter is not to make a case for palpation (see my forthcoming book "The Magic Hand Returns Spring, The Art of Palpatory Diagnosis"). However, it has been observed that palpation, which can show physical and subtle energy states in the body, is becoming a lost Chinese art. Proper palpation of Neiguan, for example, can be a reliable indicator, not only of health but of stagnation and of any disharmonies that would result if PC 6 is "not doing its job."

One indispensable and impressive argument for the importance of point palpation in determining pathology comes from H. C. Dung, M.D., of the Departments of Anatomy and Physical Medicine and Rehabilitation at the University of Texas Health Science Center, San Antonio. According to Dr. Dung, points have three functional stages that could be called the status or health of a point. These functional phases have different clinical manifestations depending on the state of bodily health or the energetics they represent. These stages—active, passive, and latent—are discussed below.[4]

Points are active when the provinces that they dominate or manage are diseased. Examples would include a headache characterized by a drilling pain at GB 20 (Fengchi), sinus pressure at BL 2 (Zanzhu) or ST 2 (Sibai), itchy palms at HT 8 (Shaofu) following an allergic reaction, or pinpoint chest tightness at CV 17 (Tanzhong). Active points are indeed active: they shout for help, their voices rising to consciousness, screaming for attention with the cry of, "Help, I am diseased."

Passive points are points that become active only under mechanical processes such as palpation, electropoint detection, or other physical means. The reason they respond to such probing is that a diseased state is underway in the functional aspect of the organ-meridian complex that each point represents. They are not clamoring for attention through the spontaneous firing of nerves that evoke pain. However, their tenderness on pressure signifies what could be called the presymptomatic, preprodromal aspects of a syndrome.

The clinical significance of passive points cannot be overstated. It is their pathology as evidenced by an ah shi (Oh, yes!) response on the part of the patient that suggests energetic imbalances in the body. These imbalances may lead to more overt, quantitative, measurable, concretized diseases in the future. In general, the earlier a "dis-ease" or pattern of disharmony can be identified, the more favorable the prognosis.

Any point can fall into the category of a passive point. By definition, what makes a point passive is that it lies quiet until explored in some manner. Traditionally, certain categories of points in Chinese medicine have been described as potentially passive points. Therefore, some writers recommend that some if not all points actually be palpated as part of a Chinese physical exam. Each category of points, be it Front Mu (Alarm

---

4. Dung HC: Characterization of the three functional phases of acupuncture points. *Chi Med J*, 1984; 97(10): 751–754.

points), Back Shu (Associated points), Yuan (Source points), Xi (cleft) (points of accumulation or blockage), or clinically effective points (points with known diagnostic and treatment values), presides over a domain that can refer to various conditions in the body. Yet any point can be a passive point and can be adopted by the practitioner to verify the diagnosis. Because of the multiplicity of roles that PC 6 (Neiguan), plays in the body, it becomes both an important indicator of the pathology or health of what the point covers, as well as being a significant point in treatment.

Finally, Dr. Dung proposes a category of points known as latent points. Latent points are inactive points that neither fire spontaneously nor are stimulated to the level of pain through mechanical means. Palpation of latent points may produce the typical sensations of qi arrival: heat, numbness, distention, redness, electrical or other sensation radiating to a particular area. However, by interacting with the patients and carefully observing them, the practitioner should be able to discern the difference between pain, the absence of a response, or qi arrival caused by stimulating the inherent healthy energy of a point. Obviously, the more latent points the body has, the healthier it is. The lack of pain felt by the patient or the lack of tension, tightness, or mushiness perceived by the practitioner indicates the functional integrity of the Inner Gate.

In short, in the most ideal situation, PC 6 is a latent point and in the healthy person this is borne out. However, if any of the roles that Neiguan plays are impaired, there are varying degrees of tenderness at this site. Clinically, PC 6 on the left side in both men and women seems to be the most reliable indicator of point dysfunction. Various sources have suggested that PC 6 should be used on the right in women and on the left in men because of the correspondence of yin/yang with gender. However, eight years of treatment on hundreds of patients have revealed that the left-sided Neiguan is more effective for both sexes. The reason for this seems to be that each organ-meridian complex has a particular left-right affinity that is expressed in many of the historical pulse systems summarized in *Table 33* and illustrated in *Figure 17*.

*Table 33.* An Historical Comparison of Various Pulse Diagnosis Systems

| Pulse Systems | Position | RIGHT HAND | | | LEFT HAND | | |
|---|---|---|---|---|---|---|---|
| | | Distal | Middle | Proximal | Distal | Middle | Proximal |
| *Yellow Emperor's Classic (Neijing)* ca. 200 B.C. | superficial deep | Chest LU | SP ST | abdomen KI | sternum HT | diaphragm LR | abdomen KI |
| *Five Element Classic (Nanjing)* ca. 200 B.C. | superficial deep | LI LU | ST SP | TE PC | SI HT | GB LR | BL KI |
| *Wang Shu-he: Pulse Classic* ca. 280 B.C. | superficial deep | LI LU | ST SP | TE MM* | SI HT | GB LR | BL KI |
| *Li Shi-zhen: Pulse Diagnosis* A.D. 1564 | middle | LU | SP | MM* and LI TE | HT | LR | MM,* SI, BL |
| *Zhang Jie-bing: Complete Book* A.D. 1624 | superficial deep | sternum LU | ST SP | TE, MM,* SI, KI | PC HT | GB LR | BL, LI KI |
| Eight Principle Pulse system | superficial deep | LU - | ST SP | - KI yang | HT - | GB LR | - KI yin |
| Contemporary China based on the classics | superficial deep | LI, chest LU | ST SP | LI, TE, MM* | PC HT | GB LR | SI, BL KI |

Most pulse systems indicate that the energetics of the Heart, Pericardium, Liver, and Kidney tend to be relatively left-sided. The energetics of the Lung, Spleen, and Stomach have always been considered as right-sided. We can infer that because each organ-meridian complex seems to be more expressed on one side of the body, palpation as well as needling points on these meridians, may be performed unilaterally. This approach not only fosters an economy of probing and needling, but more significantly denotes the most clinically effective points.

Previously, I pointed out that one of the most im-

*\*MM: Mingmen (Gate of Life) = Kidney yin and yang, immutably bound together*
*Source: International Training Center of the Academy of Traditional Chinese Medicine, Beijing, 1988, 1989.*

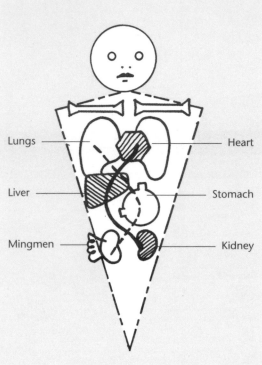

*Figure 17.* Energy Crosses

portant functions of Neiguan in the body is to be the Inner Pass,[5] the Inner Gate that can meter internal stagnation, among other things. Mark D. Seem in his most recent book, *Acupuncture Imaging, Perceiving the Energy Pathways of the Body,*[6] points out an important treatment principle of traditional Chinese medicine. He reminds us that when we free local obstructions by dispersing blockages at the surface, both the therapist and the client become more aware of the patient's constitution or body-mind, energetic core. Because true excesses in the body are actually rare (and are more likely a result of underlying deficiencies), treatment strategies can become complicated. However, if we accept the relationship of PC 6 to stagnation and the hypotheses expounded earlier (that PC 6 may be *the* best point with which to assess stagnation in the body, and the high value of palpation as both a tool of diagnosis and treatment), the use of PC 6 (Neiguan) appears imperative as the vehicle for getting qi in motion. Thus, the root cause of both stagnation and the underlying deficiencies may be rectified.

## Treatment Techniques

I have established the multiple values of PC 6 (Neiguan) as a diagnostic point. Now I want to discuss the treatment of the conditions it conjures up. Two major avenues come to mind—palpation and needling.

Palpation can be a method of treatment in its own right; however, it has treatment benefits that exceed the

5. Acupoints Research Committee of China, Society of Acupuncture and Moxibustion: *Brief Explanation of Acupoints of the 14 Regular Meridians.* Kai Z (trans). Beijing, PRC, 1987; p 77.

6. Seem MD: *Acupuncture Imaging, Perceiving the Energy Pathways of the Body.* Healing Arts Press, Rochester, Vt., 1990; p 85.

scope of this article. But I want to reiterate Dr. Van Nghi's contention that when a point is located correctly and its qi is contacted, issues of method (needling, palpation), whether to use the point bilaterally or unilaterally, the time element, and other variables become insignificant. Palpation clearly can move things, as well as bring energy to an area and this is certainly the case for PC 6.

Needling any point following palpation further reinforces the therapeutic action of the point—it secures it, "pins it down," if you will. Other variables may determine whether PC 6 or any other point simply needs to be palpated or needled. The use of these other techniques depends on the practitioner's assessment of each case, his or her own abilities, the preferred diagnostic paradigms, and other factors that are impossible to elucidate here. *Table 34* below lists the techniques that can be applied to Neiguan as one of the fundamental points of treatment.

*Table 34.* Treatment Schematic for PC 6 (Neiguan)

| Point | PC 6 (Neiguan), left side |
|---|---|
| Location | Two cun proximal to the transverse crease of the wrist, between the tendons of the m. palmaris longus and m. flexor carpi radialis |
| Palpation technique and sensation | Firm perpendicular palpation with thumb about one cun deep toward TE 5 (Waiguan). Patient will feel a mild ache to a very strong electrical sensation if the disease is subclinical to overtly manifest, respectively. To the practitioner the point may feel tense, tendinous, with very tight spacing between the tendons, indicative of qi stagnation; or mushy with loose spacing between the tendons, indicating Liver blood deficiency. |
| Needling technique | With a #1 or 36-gauge needle, insert superficially and perpendicularly .3–.5 cun. Obtain a slight to great amount of qi (depending upon the diagnosis and sensation of deficiency or excess, respectively, patient constitution, and condition.) As qi can arrive quickly at this point, search for it slowly. Perform tonification or dispersion. Sensation will range from mild to strong distention or numbness, spreading from PC 6 distally to the middle finger or proximally to the elbow or armpit. |

# Patient Education and Empowerment

Neiguan is very easy to locate and stimulate. Therefore, if it is either an active point (rare) or a passive point (very common—about 75 percent of the time), patients can be shown how to regulate their own internal conditions by rubbing this point.

Firm, deep, dispersive pressure can be applied by the patient several times daily. As the patient learns to correlate the tension at the point with clinical manifestations that suggest stagnation such as tension headaches, period cramping, nausea, chest tightness, emotional upset, irritability, stomach upset, and fainting, to name a few, the treatment can be used as needed. More gentle rubbing of the point distally toward the fingers can be done if the point sensation on palpation is achy or feels mushy. This technique can also be used simply because the patient likes it (indicative of deficiency). The treatment strengthens the emptiness of the essential substances that this palpatory confirmation suggests; it improves immunity and supplements the body with ancestral qi.

Such self-treatment accelerates the therapeutic process and clears patterns of disharmony so that the practitioner can perform the treatments that are difficult or impossible for patients to administer. Equally, if not more importantly, patients can learn more about their bodily energetics so they can assume responsibility for them. Considerable medical knowledge can be given to the average person instead of being held exclusively by medical experts. In this way, patients are greatly empowered to help themselves. Also, they are more likely to comply with educational prescriptives when they are actively involved in the therapeutic process instead of being mysteriously "fixed." And the practitioner fulfills the early *Neijing* maxim to doctors that "the superior physician is a teacher"—certainly a noble pursuit.

## Conclusions

I have explored a schematic outline and theoretical justification for the use of PC 6 (Neiguan) so that practitioners can add to or review their repertoire of skills. What I hope I have conveyed in this chapter is the preeminence of the clinical significance of PC 6 (Neiguan) and how to use it both in diagnosis and in treatment as the criterion or gauge of internal well-being. In addition, I have emphasized palpation as the modality that both diagnoses and redresses illness. Furthermore, there are other treatment strategies—such as moving stagnation, clearing excesses, and providing patient education—so that the inner barrier[7] can be maintained. Indeed, the gate to our inner well-being is just within our reach, thanks to the wisdom of the human body and the sagacity of Chinese medicine, at the site of the Inner Gate, PC 6.

7. Darras JC: *Traite D'Acuponcture Medicale,* Tome I. Barnett M (trans). O.I.C.S. Newsletter, 1982; 23.

# THE TREATMENT OF DISEASE WITH SPECIFIC PROTOCOLS

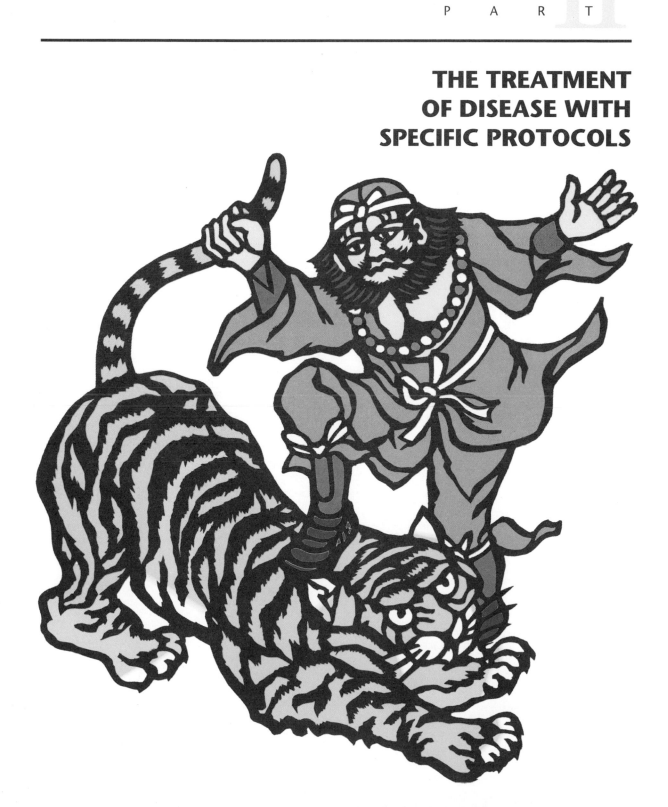

# THE TREATMENT OF PERIODONTAL GUM DISEASE
## A Protocol for Prevention, Maintenance, and Reversal Within the Paradigm of Classical Chinese Medicine

Periodontal gum disease is a degenerative disorder that affects millions of Americans and undoubtedly many more millions world wide. Western medicine and dentistry, with most of its therapy confined to oral surgery once the disease has progressed to an advanced stage, has limited success. On the other hand, classical Chinese medicine, with its characteristic approach of perceiving the body in terms of relationships, explains gum problems as stemming from organ disharmonies, in particular those of the Stomach and Spleen. This unique framework offers an alternative and effective therapeutic approach with more successful results. More importantly, the classical Chinese methods offer ways to prevent this pathology from developing in the first place.

## Etiology, Pathogenesis, and Prognosis in Western Medicine

Periodontal gum disease—a progression of gingivitis to the point of losing the supporting bone of the teeth—is the primary cause of tooth loss in over seventy-five million adult Americans. It may begin as early as age fifteen in young adults and by age sixty-five has claimed some teeth in virtually everyone.[1]  Its etiology is identical to the same local and systemic factors responsible for its precursor, gingivitis:  an inflammation of the tissues that surround and support the teeth.

According to the *Merck Manual*,[2] the leading cause of this illness is poor dental hygiene, which generally consists of improper brushing and lack of periodic, professional cleaning.  Both of these can remove bacterial microorganisms known as plaque that attach themselves to the teeth and can become calcified and are then identified as calculus or tartar.  Secondary factors include mouth breathing, food impaction, faulty dental restorations, and/or occlusion of the jaw (which causes an excess load to be carried by the teeth).  According to Western medicine, gingivitis can be the first sign of a systemic disorder such as diabetes, leukemia, or vitamin deficiency.  The skilled practitioner should be acquainted with these differentiating signs and symptoms.

Unless the causative factor is systemic, in which case those reasons need to be addressed, the treatment of gingivitis generally centers around improving dental hygiene.  This strategy can be both effective and sufficient if followed.  However, if gingivitis advances to periodontitis, pockets begin to develop between the teeth and become places where food and microorganisms can collect and proliferate.  The teeth then become detached from the gums and bone loss begins.  Unless an acute problem is superimposed upon a chronic one, pain is generally absent.  At this point, oral surgery is the recommended course of action according to dentists, an approach that is not only expensive and traumatic, but also in many cases is only palliative.

1. *Periodontal Diseases—Don't Wait Till It Hurts*.  American Dental Association, Chicago, 1992.

2. Berlow R (ed):  *The Merck Manual*.  Merck and Company, Inc., Rahway, N.J., 1987; pp 2333–2334.

# Etiology, Pathogenesis, and Prognosis in Classical Chinese Medicine

Because of the descriptions of organ interrelationships in Chinese medicine, we have no problem understanding how gingivitis and periodontitis could be manifestations of a systemic disorder. However, the etiology or root cause of this malady is usually an affliction of one particular organ-meridian complex: the Stomach and the factors that contribute to Stomach disharmonies.

According to zang-fu theory, the Stomach organ-meridian complex opens to the mouth and its health is reflected in the mucous membranes of the oral cavity, including the gums. When gingival tissue becomes red, inflamed, ulcerated with bleeding, and the breath is bad, as in the case of gingivitis, this condition in Chinese medicine is termed "Heat in the Stomach," "Blazing Stomach Fire," or "Hyperactivity of the Fire of the Stomach" because of the obvious symptoms of heat-fire in the Stomach. Hence, all the conditions that can lead to Stomach heat-fire are involved in this ailment, although some are more common than others. At times the Spleen may become involved if the heat in the Stomach makes the blood hot, thereby causing extravasation of blood from the vessels. For easy reference, these etiological factors and the mechanisms by which such manifestations mature are summarized in *Table 35*.

*Table 35.* Factors Contributing to Stomach Heat and Periodontal Gum Disease

| ETIOLOGICAL FACTORS | MECHANISMS |
|---|---|
| **FOOD** | |
| 1. Ingestion of energetically hot foods into the Stomach either in excess or in excess relative to the patient. The most common offenders are hot, spicy, pungent foods, e.g., chili, curry, red meat, chocolate, sugar, and other acidic foods. | 1. Direct entry of hot foods into the Stomach, causing it to overheat. |
| 2. Overeating of damp foods that are difficult for the Spleen and Stomach to break down, e.g., dairy products, greasy, damp, oily, or rich foods. | 2. When the Spleen fails to transform and transport the digesta, stagnation may ensue. Stagnation frequently transforms into heat and/or fire, which serves to perversely heat up the middle jiao. |
| **ALCOHOL** | |
| One of the greatest offenders, especially wine (Evil Wetness) or other "hot" alcoholic beverages, e.g., whiskey, tequila. | Causes heat in the Stomach either directly or by virtue of the failure of the Spleen to transform and transport. |
| **STRESS** | |
| Most stress is indicative of the inability of the Liver qi to flow freely. | When Liver qi stagnates for any reason, it may overact on the earth element causing Spleen qi to become deficient and Stomach qi to ascend and oftentimes heat up. |
| **DENTAL HYGIENE** | |
| Improper brushing or failure to brush teeth, lack of flossing and/or insufficient professional visits to correct the oral environment through cleaning, scraping, and other recommended dental procedures. | Lack of proper dental hygiene causes plaque to proliferate in the mouth, leading to Stomach heat or buildup of calcified plaque that further leads to gum and bone erosion. |

# A Comprehensive Protocol for the Prevention, Maintenance, and Reversal of Periodontal Gum Disease

The treatment and prevention of gingival and periodontal gum disease can be approached by addressing the etiological factors highlighted in *Table 35*. This can be done especially by altering the diet, improving dental hygiene, and reducing stress, depending on which patterns are most prevalent.

In response to this profile, I have devised the Gardner-Abbate Periodontal Protocol (GAPP) for the prevention, maintenance, and reversal of gum problems. Steps 1 through 11 of this protocol emphasize dental hygiene. They were devised in 1978, based on doctors' recommendations, research, and clinical experience, and have proven to be reliable. Steps 12 through 15 were added to the protocol between 1981 and 1984 and represent an Oriental treatment strategy. Poor dental practices can still be subsumed under Stomach heat because of the mouth's connection with the Stomach and the nature of the microorganisms, acidity, and food impaction, which can be viewed as pathogens leading to Stomach heat. Steps 16 through 17 are imperative to achieve compliance and the favorable results that this protocol can produce. This protocol is summarized below in *Table 36*.

*Table 36.* The Gardner-Abbate Periodontal Protocol (GAPP)

| | |
|---|---|
| 1. | Brush teeth every morning and evening |
| 2. | Use the Butler Stimulator |
| 3. | Floss teeth |
| 4. | Rinse with liquid chlorophyll and water |
| 5. | Brush with baking soda |
| 6. | Apply a paste of baking soda and hydrogen peroxide to the gums |
| 7. | Rinse with a salt water solution |
| 8 | Apply IPSAB® tincture to the gums |
| 9. | Have teeth cleaned and gums scraped professionally every three months |
| 10. | Take blood cleansers |
| 11. | Eat one or two pieces of fresh fruit daily |
| 12. | Avoid food and factors that lead to Stomach heat (see Table 35) |
| 13. | Take appropriate herbal prescriptions |
| 14. | Reduce stress |
| 15. | Receive acupuncture once a week |
| 16. | Believe in the body's capacity to heal itself |
| 17. | Follow the protocol exactly |

In using this protocol, patients fell into two groups: those who complied and those who did not. There has been a 100 percent success rate for those patients who have complied with the program. In the next section of this chapter, actual cases are discussed and the reasons for noncompliance are outlined.

## A. Dental Procedures

## (Note: Perform steps 1 through 9 in this order.)

1. To rid the mouth of bacteria that have built up overnight, brush the teeth properly every morning. Repeat in the evening before going to bed. Angle the head of the toothbrush against the gum line with short strokes (about half a tooth wide) and move the brush back and forth several times using a gentle scrubbing motion.[3] A soft nylon bristle brush is suggested instead of a hard bristle brush. Improper brushing and natural boar bristles, for example, may actually damage the gums, enlarge gum pockets, and be an idiopathic source of the problem. It is preferable to use a nonsweetened, nonfluoride toothpaste. Fluoride can cause tooth mottling (discoloration), especially in high doses. More poisonous than lead and slightly less poisonous than arsenic, it may be that even in low doses the fluoride ion is toxic. As a rule, natural toothpastes such as those found in health food stores are good choices.

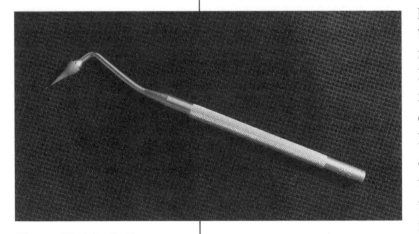

***Figure 18.*** The Butler G-U-M® Stimulator

2. With an implement called the Butler G-U-M® Stimulator *(Figure 18)*, position the rubber tip on the gums between each tooth space; press downward and from side to side. The pressure from this action drains gum capillaries, promotes improved blood circulation to the affected area, and firms up the gums. The metal Butler stimulator can be purchased at most supermarkets or pharmacies. The rubber end on some toothbrush handles is not adequate

---

3. *Caring for your teeth and gums.* American Dental Association, Chicago, 1994.

because it does not have the metal base underneath the rubber tip to provide adequate pressure for this critical massage.

3. Floss the teeth correctly every evening, gently moving the floss away from the gum by scraping up and down against the side of each tooth.[4]  The goal is to clean the teeth and stimulate the gums. Unwaxed floss seems to clean better, although waxed floss can be effective, especially for closely spaced teeth.  Do not cut the gums by using the floss incorrectly in a seesaw motion.

4. Rinse the mouth with a solution of liquid chlorophyll and water—about one teaspoon of chlorophyll to three ounces of water.  Vigorously swish the mixture around in the mouth and do not swallow. Liquid chlorophyll can be purchased at health food stores in the refrigerated department, or wheat grass juice, a rich source of chlorophyll, can be substituted.  The chlorophyll oxygenates the gums.  Because of their ingredients and alcohol content, I never recommend the use of commercial mouthwashes.

5. Brush the teeth again by dipping the toothbrush into a dime-size amount of  baking soda.  Being alkaline, it neutralizes an acidic mouth, the breeding ground of many plaque- and tartar-causing microorganisms.  Baking soda also removes the green stain left by the chlorophyll.

6. In the palm of the hand make a small paste of baking soda and hydrogen peroxide and spread on the gums.  Leave in place for approximately three minutes and avoid swallowing the mixture.  This step assists in oxygenating the gums, a function seen by the little bubbles in the area.

---

4. *Caring for your teeth and gums.*

7. Mix about a half teaspoon of salt, preferably sea salt, to three ounces of warm water. Rinse the mouth with this solution, which strengthens the gums and their connective tissue, and adjusts the acidity of the mouth.

8. Apply IPSAB® tincture to the gums with a cotton swab. This is an herbal treatment solution that contains prickly ash bark, sodium chloride, calcium chloride, iodine trichloride, and essence of peppermint. According to John Christopher, N.D., this liquid extract "astringes the gums and the local blood vessels thereby leading to improved gum tone and circulation to the affected area."[5] William McGarey, M.D., says that the ingredients in IPSAB® were described in the Edgar Cayce readings as a specific for destroying the bacillus that he identified as the causative factor in infection of pyorrhea (periodontitis).[6] IPSAB® can be purchased or special ordered at most large health food stores.

9. Have the teeth cleaned and gums scraped by a dental professional every three months. During the cleaning, the depth of pocket formations can be measured, and changes and progress noted. The patient should keep a copy of this chart and return it to the Oriental medical practitioner so that changes can be monitored.

## B. Dietary/Herbal Recommendations

10. Take blood cleansers, such as chlorophyll tablets, internally to assist in purifying (i.e., cooling) the blood.

11. Eat one or two pieces of fresh fruit per day. In moderation, fruit helps to cool the Stomach. The

5. Christopher J: *School of Natural Healing.* BiWorld Publishers, Inc., Provo, Utah, 1976; pp 138, 454.

6. McGarey W: *Physician's Reference Notebook.* Association for Research and Enlightenment, Virginia Beach, Va., 1968.

astringent quality of strawberries is particularly beneficial and they can be directly rubbed onto the gums as well. Chewing crunchy fruit like apples helps keep the bone from degenerating.

12. The poor dietary habits listed in *Table 35* (see Chapter Sixteen) increase the incidence of gum problems because they add heat to the Stomach, which reflects in the mouth and causes the classical signs of gum deterioration. In Chinese medicine, the mouth is described as the reflection of the Stomach, and Western physicians would agree at least that this connection exists because digestion begins in the mouth. Avoid food and drink that heats the Stomach and that results in bleeding gums and other characteristics of gingivitis and periodontitis. Ideally, eliminate these agents, especially during the recovery phase (about one year). In addition, because heat in the Stomach increases appetite, which in turn escalates Stomach heat, the appetite needs to be curbed by consciously decreasing the amount of food and monitoring the food intake.

13. Herbal formulas can greatly help to resolve the disease. Formulas, like acupoints, should be selected depending on the syndrome differentiation. However, there are several excellent formulas that have great clinical utility, specifically, Brion's freeze-dried products. Three that I have used with good result are detailed below.

    a) Cinnamon Five-Herb Combination (Kuei-chih-wu-wu-tang or Gui Zhi Wu Wu Tang) is perhaps the formula of choice because of its broad range of action on oral illness. This formula improves blood circulation in the upper part of the body (e.g., mouth and gums), reduces swelling, relieves moist heat (e.g., damp-heat from alcohol consumption), dispels internal heat (e.g., of the

Stomach), and nourishes the Spleen.

b) Rhubarb Five-Herb Combination (Wu-wu-ta-huang-tang) is indicated if inflammation is the predominant complaint as it is in the case of gingivitis. This formula clears heat, removes toxicity, activates circulation, and moves blood stagnation.

c) Pueraria Combination (Ko-ken-tang) is beneficial at the very onset. Energetically, the formula improves circulation, strengthens gastrointestinal function and has a detoxifying action on the liver.[7] Chinese herbal patent medicines and freeze-dried formulations seem to enhance patient compliance because they are easy to take. Tinctures with an alcohol base are generally contraindicated in this illness because of their inherent heat. As many practitioners know, decoctions tend to be too time consuming for most American patients although they can be very effective. Depending on the complexity of the patient's condition, herbal evaluations should be performed weekly when the patient comes for acupuncture. However, the formulas we have suggested can usually be prescribed and taken for a one-month period and evaluated at that time for appropriateness, dosage, side effects, and therapeutic effectiveness.

## C. Lifestyle Changes

14. Reduce stress through exercise and/or deep relaxation. Ten to twenty minutes of exercise per day is extremely beneficial in curtailing the Liver from overacting on the earth element, another mechanism by which the Stomach can become hot and

---

7. Hsu H-Y (ed): *Natural Healing with Chinese Herbs.* Oriental Healing Arts Press, Los Angeles, 1982; p 542.

the Spleen deficient (see *Table 35*).

15. Acupuncture administered once a week is ideal. With this therapy the patient receives energetic support during the initial three- or four-month period, the most critical phase during which new habits can be established, questions clarified, and organ physiology stabilized and returned to normal. Tongue, pulse, and palpation can physically verify changes. This feedback is both encouraging to the patient and indispensable to the practitioner. Select the points based upon the symptoms that the patient presents and that translate into a pattern of syndrome differentiation.

    Various sources can be consulted for specific, clinically effective points. However, my inclination is not to prescribe point formulas but to treat the patient *as a unique configuration of energy*. There is, however, one acupoint that stands out as perhaps the quintessential point to verify the degree of Stomach heat. That point is an Extra point opposite the location of ST 44 (Inner Neiting, Inner Court). This Extra point is located on the sole of the foot between the second and third toes at the junction of the margin of the web, hence the name Lineiting ("Within the Inner Court"). If heat is present, this point tends to be more tender on the right foot due to the affinity of certain organs for one side of the body or the other. Patients should be taught how to press this point firmly on a daily basis to stimulate the inherent power of ST 44 (Inner Neiting) as the water point that helps cool the Stomach.

16. Encourage the patient to believe in the body's capacity to heal itself. This mind set, a mental form of qi, raises the qi and helps it to circulate in its proper pathway.

17. Encourage the patient to impeccably follow the protocol.

# Clinical Experience: Success and Limitations

In terms of reducing the size of periodontal pockets or at least maintaining the initial measurements, positive results should be seen by a dentist or dental hygienist in three to four months. When dental professionals say that surgery is needed and then start to see changes as a result of this or other programs, they usually do not know how to respond. From their perspective, the poor prognosis for periodontal disease reflects their education and experience. However, when dentists witness significant changes such as reduced inflammation, no bleeding, decreased redness, improved gum tone, absence of infection, curtailed bone loss (or even regeneration), reduced pocket formation, and an overall improved oral environment, they have encouraged and referred patients to continue to manage their condition through Oriental medical guidance.

Among patients who have followed this protocol, I have observed a 100 percent success rate in stopping further progression, if not actually mitigating the problem. Regeneration of the gums and reduced pocket size has been confirmed by their dentists. It takes about one year to accomplish these results, with continued progress being noted during periodic dental visits at three-, six-, nine-, and twelve-month intervals. After six months steps 4 to 9 can usually be eliminated from the dental protocol and food indulgences *in moderation* can be resumed if necessary.

Compliant patients are generally particularly adverse to the idea of surgery, not just because of fear, but more significantly because these patients tend to be open to the capacity of the body to heal itself. Therefore, patient education regarding the effects of diet, stress, and dental hygiene is a valuable part of encouraging compliance with this protocol. Practitioners should continually educate their patients about food, stress, and dental hygiene, and include the use of written handouts to reinforce their advice. The fears and insecurities that patients have can be allayed by telling them about successful cases; this also motivates them.

Noncompliant patients—those who have rejected or not adhered to the protocol—have consistently said that they were not interested in reducing alcohol consumption, changing dietary preferences, or cultivating careful dental habits. Even at the cost of surgery, they often prefer to "be fixed" rather than to assume responsibility for part of the healing process. Even after the expense, pain, and trauma of surgery, it is unfortunate but not surprising to find that the problem frequently recurs.

*Cases 13 - 16* are offered to demonstrate the use of the GAPP protocol as well as the reasons for successful and unsuccessful cases.

**Cases 13–16.** Periodontal gum disease

**Case 13.**

The patient was a forty-one-year-old female. Her major complaints were periodontal gum disease characterized by pain and inflammation, along with emotional distress at the prospect of six recommended surgeries. Symptoms of the distress included depression, inactivity, indecisiveness, lethargy, and lack of focus but lots of ideas. In addition to a hearty appetite, she reported extreme thirst. She craved buttery food, cheese, chocolate, generally rich foods, and liked food cooked in wine. She ate peanut butter daily and as a child, she had eaten "lots" of dairy foods. For five years she smoked two packs of cigarettes and drank two to three glasses of wine a day. She had also overeaten for the previous three years, gaining thirty-five pounds very rapidly.

Her tongue was reddish purple, redder on the sides and the tip. The tongue had no coat, was wet and swollen (height-wise), otherwise thin, quivery, with "thorns" or *ci* (indicating hyperactivity of pathogenic heat) in the Kidney area. She felt hot to the touch and the pulses were deficient and thin with slipperiness in the Stomach/Spleen positions.

Acupuncture treatment was administered approximately one time per week for eight months to supplement two deep cleanings from the dentist. Patient compliance was excellent in terms of weekly acupuncture treatments but poor in terms of taking herbs; compliance was also high in terms of exercise recommendations but particularly poor in eliminating wine for cooking and drinking. Exacerbating factors were clearly her food, alcohol, and prior smoking habits. After following the protocol for eight months (to the extent described), her dentist confirmed that surgery was no longer required. She was free from pain, inflammation, and had regained direction and focus in her life. Although she had avoided the need for surgery, she still needs to improve her diet and be meticulous with the dental protocol for the results to hold. Excessive alcohol use may cause the problem to resurface.

## Case 14.

The patient was a sixty-year-old female with diagnosed gum disease of ten years' duration for which she had received no dental treatment. She did not like to brush her teeth because of sensitive spots and therefore generally did not. She felt that the condition of her mouth was affecting her health and draining her energy. Other symptoms included osteoporosis, SAD (Seasonal Affective Disorder), and an impaired immune system as shown by constant viral and other infections. When she first came for a consultation, she had coincidentally suffered a severe reaction to a flu shot, with symptoms of serial otosis and agonizing facial and ear pain.

The pain reaction to the flu shot further exacerbated her aversion to touch and to brushing her teeth. Before I could treat the periodontal disease, I gave treatment for the acute symptoms from the flu shot reaction. The results were successful. In addition, the patient was able to ward off colds, which she attributed to the acupuncture and the prescribed herbs. (We cannot eliminate the possible positive effect of the flu shot, however). Prior to treatment she had had three major viral infections.

Unfortunately, she abandoned treatment, the protocol, and even brushing her teeth. She only attempted to follow the protocol once or twice because of "the devastating symptoms of SAD," which she claimed had overwhelmed her.

## Case 15.

The patient was a seventy-three-year-old male with an established diagnosis of gum deterioration, bleeding gums, tooth sensitivity to cold, and looseness and separation of the teeth. He preferred Mexican food; he had a strong appetite and drank one glass of wine every day. His dentist had recommended gum surgery.

After one week of using the dental protocol, taking Cinnamon Five-Herb Combination, and avoiding wine and spicy foods (much to his displeasure), he reported that his gums were bleeding less. Three weeks later he reported that his mouth felt better; there was less bleeding and less tooth sensitivity. He also had substantially reduced his spicy food intake.

After another three weeks his mouth continued to "feel good" with no adverse symptoms to report. One month later, after having used only the protocol (because he did not like or respond to acupuncture), his dentist's chart noted "improvement." The loose teeth were tighter and the oral hygiene appeared good. Surgery was no longer recommended by the dentist and the patient was released from my care confident that his minor dietary changes and improved oral practices could help him at least maintain his gums without the prospect of surgery. He has maintained this condition now for nearly four years.

## Case 16.

A forty-seven-year-old male patient had been told twelve years earlier that all his lower teeth would be gone by now. He had had all the prep work done for gum surgery, but a friend recommended that he see what Chinese medicine could do for him, even at this late juncture.

His symptoms of periodontal gum disease were quite advanced. They included bone loss, gum recession, bleeding gums, loose teeth, and pronounced sensitivity to extremes in temperature. The patient's diet consisted of about half raw foods and the other half cooked. He was fully aware that he consumed a pound of sugar each week. Although there is a long history of alcoholism in the family and the patient does drink alcohol on a weekly basis, he does not suffer from alchoholism.

*continued*

The major pathologies in the pulse were Stomach and Kidney yin deficiency and some slipperiness in general. This was supported by the large cavernous cracks in the tongue in the Stomach and Kidney area and a thick, yellow, greasy coat overall.

The patient did not want to spend much money for treatment, so the minimal number of treatments that I could administer was planned over the course of three months. In my experience this is enough time in which to assess the results of treatment for periodontal gum problems, and also the patient was scheduled for a dental checkup at the end of that period.

Acupuncture supplemented by herbs was the primary treatment modality and the periodontal protocol oulined above was taught to the patient. He was not interested in any dietary changes to improve the health of the Stomach and its reflection in the mouth.

After five treatments the patient reported that his teeth had tightened and his mouth was free from plaque. He had little tartar and his teeth were less sensitive to heat. His mouth felt cleaner and he felt good in general. The mobility of the lower teeth was significantly less and the gum bleeding was reduced. The dentist confirmed all of these results. As well, the Kidney pulses had significantly improved and the tongue coating had diminished.

His dentist reported that periodontal surgery was no longer necessary. I advised the patient to continue with the protocol and to return for visits if the symptoms resurfaced. In a follow-up study, I have determined that for over three years the patient has remained free of the need for oral surgery.

In summary, because of the unique perspective of classical Chinese medicine, an alternative treatment strategy to surgery for gingivitis and periodontal gum disease can be offered. As is characteristic of this paradigm, the identification and treatment of the root instead of just the symptoms gives the most enduring therapeutic effects. An added benefit to the protocol is that it can open doors to communication between Oriental and Western healthcare practitioners for the benefit of the patient. This approach contributes as well to a better understanding of the disease's etiology, pathogenesis, and prognosis.

The combined methods of better dental hygiene (which is not antithetical to the Chinese view of Stomach heat) and changing how one lives (which, in many cases, is the source of the imbalances called disease) offer some hope, or at least an option, to escape surgery.

# 16

# THE ETIOLOGY AND TREATMENT OF CELLULITE ACCORDING TO CHINESE MEDICINE
## More Than Skin Deep

Cellulite—subcutaneous deposits of fat that dimple the buttocks and limbs—is a condition that affects millions of women of all ages. Although its treatment and removal is usually confined to the beauty industry and to cosmetic surgery, its etiology and clinical significance is "more than skin deep."

*Cellulite* is considered to be a nontechnical term for such deposits of fat and therefore it is not found in most medical dictionaries. In spite of the fact that the condition is not medically defined, however, it continues to appear as lumps and dimpling on the buttocks, thighs, legs, and arms of women worldwide. Cellulite is not the exclusive domain of American women, or of overweight individuals. Aestheticians and physicians have observed that slim women are as likely (or more) to develop the "orange-peel" dimpling on the skin that characterizes this complaint. Viewed with concern by many women, some claim to have acquired this condition virtually overnight.

Because the presence of cellulite is a concern to women, it has received occasional attention from the medical profession. Perhaps because the condition is not life threatening and because it is considered to be a purely cosmetic problem, physicians tend to minimize it. Correspondingly, information on the subject in the medical literature, including sources on pathology and dermatology, is scarce. When cellulite is addressed as treatable by the medical community, it is primarily in terms of its *elimination* (specifically through liposuction) in contrast to its *prevention*. This may be because its etiology is not well understood.

Poor circulation, whether in slim or overweight women, has been suggested as a causative factor. Even after a person loses weight, cellulite may not necessarily go away. This differentiation of weight loss patterns has suggested to Western healthcare practitioners that cellulite is not just "plain" fat that can be eliminated, but may represent a combination of fat and poor lymphatic circulation. Randall Roenigk, M.D., associate professor of dermatology at the Mayo Clinic in Rochester, Minnesota, is quoted as saying, ". . . cellulite is locked-in pockets of fat. [These] clumps of fat cells are stored just under the skin in honeycomb-like structures held in place by bands of fibrous tissue. As skin loses its elasticity from aging and other factors (sun exposure, smoking, excess weight), the fat clumps become more visible, creating a dimpled look."[1]

Unproven theories have been offered to the public by so-called experts in this area. These theories include the idea that a low-fat diet coupled with aerobic exercise may be helpful in the treatment of cellulite. However, the people who suggest this usually also recognize that skin structure, body type, and hormonal influences may be additional factors in the development of cellulite. These practitioners often see such conditions as not very treatable.

From the cosmetic and medical industries, numerous innovative procedures have been devised to ameliorate cellulite. Regimens that include exercise and diet

---

1. Almasi MR: The truth about cellulite. *Redbook*, June, 1994; 46.

(designed to boost metabolic processes) tend to give more effective results than liposuction, though not as immediate, of course.

From my observations and experience over the last twenty years, it appears that there is a greater chance that a more enduring effect will result when a therapy accurately identifies and addresses the *root cause* rather than the overt manifestations. However, the root is not always clearly discernible to those who attempt to correct this condition.

Numerous treatment approaches—cultural, hypothetical, personal, and clinical—can be found in women's fashion or health magazines. These specific suggestions will not be discussed here as the purpose of this chapter is to present another explanation for this phenomenon, that is a Chinese perspective. The corresponding modalities for the condition are then described.

## Cellulite: the Progression from Dampness to Organ Dysfunction

Although I agree with the Western interpretation of cellulite as a type of fat complicated with poor lymphatic circulation, I feel that the etiology of cellulite can be better explained by classical Chinese medicine, specifically through the concept of damp-phlegm. In a survey of various Oriental sources, I was unable to find any attempt to differentiate this condition. Therefore, to support the hypothesis that cellulite is a progression on a continuum from damp to phlegm, I offer the following mechanism as summarized below in *Table 37*.

*Table 37.* The Etiology of Cellulite

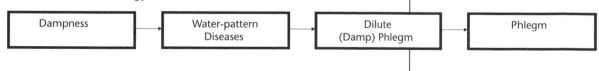

## 1. Dampness

In traditional Chinese medicine, when the Spleen fails in its role to transform and transport food and drink, dampness (*shi*), an accumulation of fluids in the Spleen, may result. Also known as pathological or evil dampness, it is by definition a secondary by-product of Spleen qi and yang deficiency. To resolve this condition there must be a dual treatment plan of transforming dampness and tonifying the qi and yang of the Spleen.

The qi of the Spleen can become deficient in many ways, the most common being a diet of rich, oily, greasy foods that are difficult for the Spleen to break down. Foods that are cold in temperature as well as energetically cold also hinder the Spleen's role in transformation and transportation because the Spleen prefers warm and dry food to fulfill its function in the body. The Spleen's energy can be further drained through emotional and lifestyle factors such as excessive work, thought, study, worry, meditation, or frequent or extended sitting, all of which compete with the Spleen's natural inclination to move or transport. Exogenous climatic dampness can also invade and weaken the Spleen, which suggests that perhaps women in damp environments would be more disposed to Spleen qi deficiency, resulting in cellulite, an interesting hypothesis that remains to be investigated. Other symptoms of Spleen qi deficiency with dampness include fatigue, abdominal distention, thin or overweight body type, poor muscle tone, feelings of heaviness, pallor, and gas. The client with cellulite commonly exhibits these symptoms.

## 2. Water-Pattern Diseases

When dampness is untreated, "water-pattern diseases" may ensue, with the most common form being edema. This water can accumulate in the upper jiao and cause facial puffiness; in the middle jiao as distention in the epigastrium; and in the lower jiao as edema that pits when pressure is applied to the affected area, displacing the accumulated water. I propose that cellulite, because of its characteristic pitted form, falls into this category.

## 3. Damp-phlegm

Unresolved "water" can become "dilute phlegm," also known as damp-phlegm (*shi tan*) or phlegm turbidity. This stage of chronic dampness is more dense and substantial, taking on a relatively more physical form. Better known clinical manifestations of damp-phlegm include mucus expectorated from the Lungs, vomiting of clear, frothy phlegm from the stomach, and edema of the limbs where the body looks swollen but has no pitting.

## 4. Phlegm

Finally phlegm, the most congealed of all of its precursors, takes many forms. Although this list is by no means complete, some of the more common forms of phlegm are kidney stones and gallstones, arthritic bone deformities, coma and mania, atherosclerosis, immovable subcutaneous nodules, and feelings of constriction in the throat.

## 5. Organ Dysfunction

It seems likely that other organ-meridian complexes involved in water processes in the body are also involved in cellulite formation, namely the Lung and the Kidney. According to classical Chinese medicine, it is the role of the Lung to control water passageways and the descent and dispersal of fluids. When this function is not performed, fluids can accumulate in the interstitial spaces of the skin, which is clearly where the cellulite surfaces.

The Kidney, as the organ mainly responsible for water metabolism, may be involved as a deeper substrate of the problem. The Kidney can fail to supplement the Spleen with the yang and warmth to do its job of transforming and transporting liquids. A Kidney association seems to be further substantiated as the retention of the damp-water entity collects in the lower jiao, distributing itself on the thighs and buttocks, where cellulite most commonly occurs.

This diagnosis of cellulite as an entity on the continuum of damp to phlegm due to a deficiency of Spleen qi and yang—sometimes complicated by deficiency of Lung and Kidney qi and yang—is consistent with the Western interpretation of cellulite, that is, trapped fat (damp) from poor circulation (yang xu).

## The Treatment of Cellulite with Chinese Modalities

If this assumption is correct, that cellulite falls somewhere along the dampness-phlegm continuum, and the Spleen, Lung, and Kidney are the primary organ complexes involved in its formation, a corresponding treatment strategy is required to deal with these etiological factors. Consequently I have developed a four-tiered approach to attack the problem. The four components of this protocol include diet, exercise, deep breathing, and massage or manual therapy. To achieve not only the best and fastest but most long-lasting results, all these elements are necessary.

### 1. Diet

As the Chinese classics remind us, the source of all dampness is the Spleen, hence an attempt to resolve dampness without considering the Spleen is fruitless. A two-pronged plan should be employed at this stage: tonify the qi and yang of the Spleen, and resolve dampness.

Foods that support the Spleen should be integrated into the diet as supplements or replacements for problematic dietary habits. Such foods are warm and dry and will check the development of dampness. Examples include well-cooked vegetables such as greens, along with yellow and orange vegetables like squash, carrots, and yams. Small amounts of eggs, dairy, fish, and chicken are allowed to provide adequate protein to support the body during this period of planned weight loss. Cooked, whole grains should be added to the diet as well. Clear, pure liquids such as spring water, fresh squeezed vegetable juices, and herb teas are necessary to flush out the tissues and nourish the body.

Bob Flaws asserts in a summary of the position of Chinese medicine about tea that moderate amounts of green tea facilitate digestion and help to reduce obesity because green tea energetically strengthens the Spleen and transforms phlegm.[2]

According to Jake Fratkin, Bojenmi Chinese Tea, ("Maintain Vigor and Grace, Reduce Fat Tea,") is an excellent, tasty, weight-loss tea. It tonifies Spleen qi and dispels fat, phlegm, and excess water. Additionally, it is associated with the removal of atherosclerotic plaque (damp-phlegm) in the blood vessels, thereby reducing the risk of high blood pressure, heart disease, and stroke.[3]

Western nutritional therapists have long recognized the benefits of barley tea as a diuretic and likewise in Chinese medicine, Coix seed (Chinese barley) performs the same function by strengthening the Spleen and promoting drainage of dampness through urination.

In an anti-cellulite regime, certain foods are mostly prohibited during the first year of body reconstruction. Frozen, canned, processed, or refined foods and drink

2. Flaws B: *Arisal of the Clear, A Simple Guide to Eating Heathy According to Traditional Chinese Medicine.* Blue Poppy Press, Boulder, Colo., 1991; pp 51–55.

3. Fratkin J: *Chinese Herbal Patent Medicines, A Practical Guide.* Institute for Traditional Medicine and Preventative Health Care, Portland, Ore., 1986; p 151. Ingredients include tea leaf, crataegus fruit, poria fungus, phaseolus seed, pogostemon, hordeum sprout, and citrus peel.

are inadvisable because of their limited, denatured value. In addition, these foods more often than not are full of chemical additives and preservatives that damage the body. Because of their damp nature, greasy fried foods and alcohol should be eliminated.

Ideally, the largest meal of the day should be at noon, with a light supper in the early evening. If necessary, snacks can include limited amounts of fresh fruit or a concentrated carbohydrate for prolonged energy. Calories should be purposely reduced for about four months to promote weight loss so that the trapped waste (damp-water) can be removed from the body.

*Table 38* lists foods that are useful for tonifying the qi and yang of the Spleen and for draining damp.[4] Foods to avoid, that is, those that overwork the Spleen and create damp, are also listed. Chinese nutritional sources such as those included in the references should be consulted for more specific ideas of what to eat. Consultation with a licensed healthcare professional can help to develop a safe dietary weight-loss plan with regard to calories.

***Table 38.*** Dietary Recommendations and Prohibitions

| **FOODS TO ENJOY** | Cooked carrots, yams, sweet potatoes, squash, turnips, pumpkin, onions, leeks, barley, corn, alfalfa, chestnuts, garlic, kidney beans, mustard greens, radishes, scallions |
|---|---|
| | Cooked whole grains, brown rice, millet, barley, whole grain breads in small amounts |
| | Cooked peaches, cherries, strawberries, dried figs, fresh ginger, cinnamon, nutmeg |
| | Small-moderate amounts of unprocessed sweeteners, such as honey, maple syrup, molasses, barley malt, rice bran syrup |
| | Small amounts of chicken, turkey, eggs, dairy, fish, cheese |
| | Small amounts of salad and fruit |
| | Small amounts of expelled pressed oils (olive, etc.) |
| | Spring water, fresh-squeezed vegetable juices, herb teas |
| | *Foods may be steamed, mashed, baked, or oil-free stir-fried (instead use water or broth). Chew well and eat in moderate amounts.* |
| **FOODS TO AVOID** | Frozen, canned, processed, and refined foods and beverages |
| | Too much fluid, too much salt |
| | Hydrogenated or partially hydrogenated oils |
| | Chilled or iced liquids |
| | Undercooked grains, tofu (not suitable for deficiency) |
| | Excessive amounts of red meat, sugar, rich foods (e.g., shellfish, pork, sardines, duck) |
| | Raw greens, asparagus, cabbage, seaweed, olives, soybeans, spinach, bok choy |
| | Oil-fried foods, alcohol |

4. Lu H: *Chinese System of Food Cures, Prevention and Remedies.* Sterling Publishing Co, Inc., New York, 1986; pp 161–174, 179–183.

## 2. Exercise

Exercise is a necessary and critical step in any effective weight-loss program. Although there is an abundance of exercise regimes, I recommend hatha yoga. This system uses various postures to support vital energy, to tone all the internal organs, invigorating and strengthening them, and to move blood and stuck energy as the body is stretched. One hour a day is ideal to cover the whole body adequately, that is, all the parts and organs. Regular practice confers not only increased stamina and endurance but promotes an incomparable feeling of well-being and physical, mental, and emotional balance. Beginners should take lessons with a hatha yoga instructor to learn the postures correctly.

## 3. Breathing

To address the Lungs as the "Master of Qi" that gives energy to all the organs, exercise and deep breathing are important in this protocol. Deep breathing (pranayama, life-force control) is an integral part of the discipline of hatha yoga. Alternatively, the client should adopt aerobic exercises to activate the heart and blood, or learn other methods of conscious, concentrated breathing, a sample of which is given here.

> *Lie flat on the back, full length, and close the eyes. Rest the hands palms up near but not touching the thighs. Start to breathe deeply and slowly through the nose, filling the lungs and causing the abdominal cavity to rise. Breathe in through the nose and out through the mouth, keeping the lower jaw relaxed. Concentrate on deep, slow, fine inhalations and exhalations. Start slowly with short sessions and then build up to and maintain this breathing for fifteen to twenty minutes. Never attempt to force the breath so that you feel strained.*

## 4. Massage or Manual Therapy

Massage is a fundamental mechanism in the removal of cellulite. Physical friction, kneading, and light pounding of the affected area on a daily basis are direct mechanical methods of increasing circulation. This is preferably done after a hot bath, shower, or in a dry sauna, which are also ways of increasing circulation. Gentle squeezing and kneading of the thighs and buttocks is most effective for people whose skin integrity is not weakened and delicate from sunlight, hormonal changes, or by constitution. Remember that patients with Spleen qi deficiency may have fragile skin and may bruise and bleed easily. In such cases, this method is contraindicated. On the other hand, the skin of the thighs is generally less vulnerable to this type of abrasion than other areas, such as the face, abdomen, and lower inner leg.

Various "cellulite creams" can be applied before the manual therapy. They lubricate and condition the skin, and make it easier to massage. Certain ingredients, particularly natural plant and seaweed extracts, seem to warm the affected area and augment circulation. Skin product manufacturers say that their anticellulite products "tone and firm" and that they have data to support such claims.

Other types of bodywork (for example, shiatsu, deep tissue massage, or a longtime staple of European skin care—lymphatic massage) administered by qualified personnel have the added benefit of promoting relaxation, improving circulation, and reducing tension. These are all necessary constituents of a body and mind that are healthy and balanced.

Light tapping with a Seven Star or Plum Blossom needle is an additional modality that reduces cellulite, the retained by-product of Spleen qi dysfunction. Use these instruments gently as minor bleeding followed by further unsightly scabbing may result. Instead of the

Plum Blossom needle, the Kung Gung hammer, also known as the "magnetic health hammer," can be used. Because the hammer does not pierce the skin, the side effects do not occur. The hammer can be used more vigorously than the Seven Star needle, thereby facilitating circulation. It can also replace the squeezing and kneading techniques previously detailed.

A simple kitchen rolling pin can also be used on the regions affected by cellulite. Starting at the knee on the inside of the thigh, repeatedly roll in an upward direction for about three minutes; only roll upward on this aspect of the thigh (along the course of the greater saphenous vein) in order to improve lower body circulation. Then, on the outer part of the thigh execute the same motion for the same length of time, but *only roll downward* from the upper part of the thigh to knee level, not below onto the softer part of the lower leg. Rolling upward may lead to headaches and other vascular disturbances. Also, do not roll below the knee on the softer part of the leg. This physical method is useful for reducing the swollen cells, assists in the breakdown of fat, and improves circulation. In my experience, inches can be lost in this way when done everyday.

Although acupuncture can certainly be used to treat deficiency of Spleen qi and yang with dampness, and point prescriptions can be easily formulated, I have chosen not to use needles but rather to use the modalities described here. The worst cases of cellulite I have treated were patients thirty to forty pounds overweight whose thighs had become misshapen from the cellulite. These cases can take between three and six months for the cellulite to disappear if the protocol is followed thoroughly. The client should be encouraged to continue with steps 1 to 3 as these are the foundation of a healthy lifestyle.

To eliminate cellulite, weight loss is expected, necessary, and desirable. Too much weight loss can be dangerous to one's health, which is one reason why a licensed healthcare physician should be consulted. Body weight can be reestablished through a revised diet of wholesome, healthy nutrients, aided by a functional Spleen/Stomach once the cellulite is eliminated.

As in all conditions, treatment success is a combination of many variables, two of which are essential: diagnostic acumen and patient compliance. Whereas statistical evidence of effectiveness may give the impression of success, what is really more important in Chinese medicine is the qualitative improvement and difference we can bring to the lives of individuals.

In summary, methodologies that match a discerning diagnosis can rectify a condition. In the case of cellulite, by using diagnostic methods from classical Chinese medicine, a problem that affects many women can be treated with results that range from improvement to complete remediation.

If we are able to see beyond its mundane manifestations, a more serious and deep-seated problem of Spleen qi deficiency with its secondary pathological product of damp are the basis of this physical abnormality. When we treat patients with this condition, we can also educate them about how to improve their bodies. This process will strengthen the earth energy and the Spleen organ-meridian complex so that the more serious sequelae of Spleen qi deficiency and dampness (for example, high cholesterol, kidney stones, atherosclerosis, and so on) do not develop. Again, the timeless wisdom of classical Chinese medicine offers us an effective lens through which to view modern problems and the restoration of health and balance.

# CHAPTER 17

# FACIAL
# REJUVENESCENCE

t is not surprising that regardless of culture, people want to improve the way they look and all too often, the affluent resort to cosmetic surgery to achieve a more youthful appearance. However, the effects of such surgery are often undesirable and painful. The inability to close the eyes completely when a face-lift is pulled too tightly is not uncommon. Over time the surgery may not hold up and can produce problems such as sagging, bloating, edema, and facial puffiness because the underlying cause of the wrinkles, that is, the root problem, was not dealt with.

In today's stressful world, it can be hard to cultivate a lifestyle in harmony with the laws of nature, but not to do so is to fight vainly the natural law. A five-step program, aimed at maintaining the body's qi and blood, will not only produce visible and supplementary effects on the complexion, the site where the health of the Heart and the vitality of the spirit is visible, but on the entire body as well.

## STEP I: Enough Sleep

This is probably the most critical step in a facial beautification program. Although the amount of sleep needed for optimum health varies with age and between individuals, a solid eight hours is required for most adults. In the Western world, sleep is not always highly valued and is frequently forfeited for entertainment, sex, work, or other activities.

From a Chinese point of view, sleep is needed to replenish the blood so that it can be purified and stored as the material basis of the spirit for daytime activities. Energetically, sleep is the period during which the spirit returns to the body instead of interacting in the daytime world. The spirit is reinvigorated and supported when its anchor, the blood, has been renewed. From a Western point of view, apart from the obvious need to rest, adequate sleep is required to facilitate the transfer of memory from short- to long-term, certainly an important reason to get enough sleep.

## STEPS II and III: Emotions and Diet

The role of regulating the emotions probably runs a close second to the importance of adequate rest for the body. If healthy emotions are viewed as qi going in its proper direction, one way of ensuring healthy emotions is to promote the health of the zang-fu organs. When the organs are healthy, they have adequate energy and they circulate that energy correctly. A nutritious diet, sound sleep, and exercise all promote sound physiological functioning, which fosters the creation of the qi and blood essential to health. These habits consequently provide the material basis for energy and its proper circulation, which benefits the body as well as the emotions.

When the body's qi and blood are ample and circulate in the way they should according to zang-fu physiology, the emotional life of the person tends to be balanced as well. Problematic emotions, which are simply qi flowing in perverse patterns, are less likely to occur when they are under physiological control, that is, when the zang-fu organs have enough qi and blood, are balanced in yin and yang, and are performing their specific physiological roles. The individual is also less likely to be affected by external environmental stimuli when the qi is properly maintained. Regulation of the emotional life is greatly enhanced by respecting the needs of the organs as well as our dietary, sleep, and exercise requirements. When the individual is healthy and the proper emotions are flowing in response to environmental stimuli, the face is animated and perverse emotions appearing as deep facial wrinkles do not develop. And if laugh lines do develop around the mouth and eyes, they express a joyous spirit; they are not necessarily undesirable wrinkles that need to be erased.

Since the focus of this book is not on nutrition, I will make only some general comments about food as it pertains to the health and beauty of the face. They are listed below; suggested reading can be found in the Bibliography (see also *Table 38*, Dietary Recommendations and Prohibitions in Chapter Sixteen).

1. Avoid caffeinated products (coffee, chocolate) that are vasoconstrictors. These substances elevate blood pressure but restrict arterial blood flow to the facial capillaries. Because they inhibit blood circulation, these substances tend to cause gray hair and a dull complexion. Also, the hot nature of these products can cause blood extravasation, which can produce broken facial capillaries.

2. Avoid excessive consumption (always relative to the person) of products that are damp and/or cold in nature (dairy, bananas, tofu, salads, uncooked food). These foods hamper the transforming and transporting ability of the Spleen, thereby decreasing blood production and resulting in the retention of turbid pathological products of damp in the body. This process leads to a "dirty" or muddy complexion.

3. Eat foods that are warm in nature (noodles, rice, vegetables, and foods that benefit the blood). They make it easier to digest and assimilate the rich nutrients that build ample blood.

# STEPS IV and V: Acupuncture and Facial Massage

1.  The Ten Needle Technique, used for any deficiency condition, aims at promoting the production of qi, blood, and yin. This needle combination, along with the use of the moxa box on the lower abdomen, further enhances the production of qi and blood. As with many acupuncture prescriptions, Ten Needle Technique can be used as a basic formula; other points that will nourish the blood and keep the Heart healthy may be added. Weekly treatments are recommended (see Chapter Ten, "Ten Needle Technique," for a discussion of this treatment strategy).

2.  If the patient has acne or facial breakouts, several approaches can be taken. One protocol is to use the points that clear heat or damp-heat in the blood. Clinically effective points include the following:

> LI 4 (Hegu). It is useful for Lung problems, such as skin disorders, and helps to eliminate heat, relieve redness and toxicity, and quiets the nerves.
>
> BL 12 (Fengmen) and BL 13 (Feishu). As the Back Shu points of the upper lungs and lungs, respectively, they control the skin.
>
> SP 10 (Xuehai). It harmonizes and cools the blood, clears heat, eliminates damp, clears wind-heat and wind-damp.
>
> LI 11 (Quchi). As the Earth point on the Metal meridian, it cools the blood.

Optional, supplemental points include the following:

> BL 40 (Weizhong) brings heat down.
>
> BL 17 (Geshu), an influential point that dominates the blood, and
>
> KI 1 (Yongquan) brings heat down and cools the blood.

3.  Another approach is to determine the meridian involved, based on the location of the eruptions.

According to this strategy, the Source point of the affected meridian and the Huatuojiaji point of the affected dermatome can be needled *(see Figure 19, Dermatome Map).*

4.  For small wrinkles, sterile intradermal needles (Spinex 3-6 millimeters) implanted for three days to a week, depending on humidity levels, are highly effective especially when the patient uses a mixture of pearl powder and Vitamin E oil, or a commercially prepared pearl cream moisturizer, on a daily basis to replenish the skin.

5.  Another effective therapy is to perform or receive on a daily or weekly basis a five-minute facial massage. The massage sequence from beginning to end is as follows:

1.  Special Point at the bridge of nose, directly below Yintang
2.  Yintang
3.  GV 23  (Shangxing)
4.  GV 20 (Baihui)
5.  ST 9 (Renying)
6.  GB 8 (Shuaiqu)
7.  GB 14 (Yangbai)
8.  Sinus massage including Yuyao and BL 2 (Zanzhu)

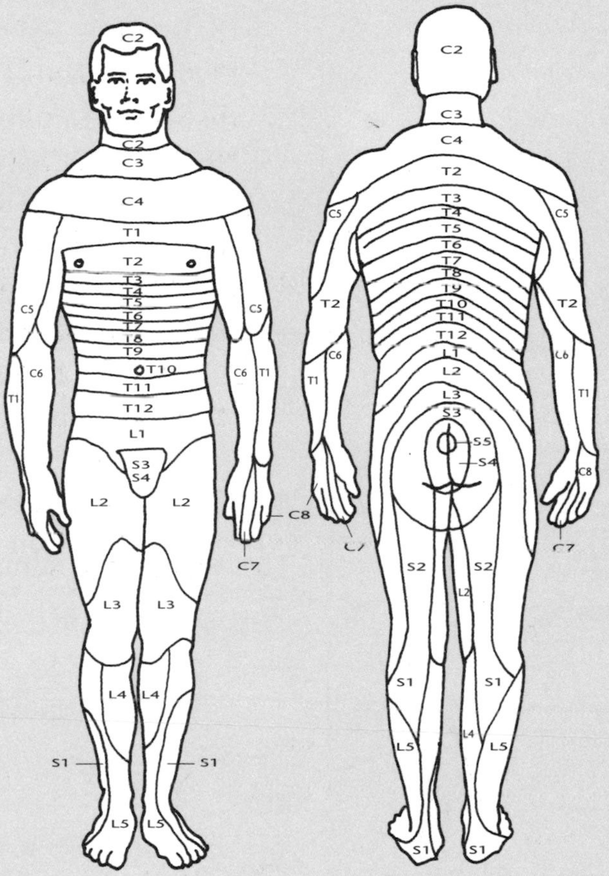

C = cervical
T = thoracic
L = lumbar
S = sacral

An area of skin whose sensory axons feed into a single dorsal root of a spinal nerve is called a dermatome. There is no universal agreement as to the precise area covered by any one dorsal root.

*Figure 19.* Dermatome Map

9. Shangming (between Yuyao and eyebrow)
10. BL 1 (Jingming)
11. LI 19 (Kouheliao)
12. LI 20 (Yingxiang)
13 Bitong
14. ST 3 (Juliao)
15. ST 4 (Dicang)
16. ST 5 (Daying)
17. ST 6 (Jiache)
18. ST 7 (Xiaguan)
19. GB 3 (Shangguan)
20. SI 18 (Quanliao)
21. CV 24 (Chengjiang)
22. Nose Heliao (directly below ST 4 and level with CV 24)
23. GV 26 (Shuigou)

This sequence is summarized in *Figure 20.* In combination, the factors of enough sleep, harmonized emotions, sound diet, acupuncture, and facial massage keep the body, mind, heart, and skin healthy and ample in qi and blood. The complexion will mirror this abundance.

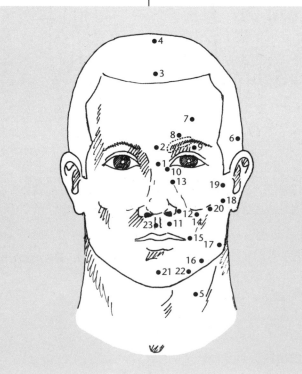

***Figure 20.*** Facial Massage Sequence

*8 = Area indicated by dashed lines*

# CHAPTER 18

# MENOPAUSE
## Mid-life Myth or
## Mirror of the Essential Substances?

**M**enopause is the cessation of a woman's menses due to decreased ovarian function. It is a biological fact of life, a natural occurrence. For over 80 percent of the female population, however, this normal event can be a physiological nightmare characterized by hot flashes, emotional aberrations, and possible osteoporosis. According to Western medical theory, the symptoms of menopause come from hormonal imbalance. Consistent with this idea, the Western physician attempts to correct this condition, usually by replacing the hormones, a therapy with considerable risks to some patients. Chinese medicine is empowered by a vision of menopause as a natural state; menopause is seen, therefore, as an expression of the qi that directs the female life cycle. This view of menopause is less problematic. To the receptive patient and the careful practitioner, menopause, like many illnesses, can be used to assess the individual's inner state, an opportunity to redress disturbances in the vital qi of the body. Menopause as a crisis can become the Chinese concept of crisis as "opportunity" if we understand the normal female life cycle, which points the way to natural correction instead of chemical intervention.

# Western Etiology and Treatment

Apart from the cessation of the menses, approximately 80 percent of women experience some degree of menopausal symptoms.  The other 20 percent experience hardly any of the symptoms that have become the hallmark of the female climacteric.  The most common psychological and physical manifestations include, but are not limited to, hot flashes, chills, mood swings, depression, irritability, insomnia, vaginal dryness, fatigue, osteoporosis, and abnormal uterine bleeding.

As ovarian function decreases, the menstrual cycle reduces in frequency and finally stops.  With decreased ovarian function there are changes with the endocrine organs such as the thyroid, hypothalamus, and kidney.  As a result, changes are likely to occur that affect the blood vessels, the nervous system, and the emotions, so that a variety of symptoms can occur.

Other women may experience what is termed premature menopause.  Premature menopause is not a function of naturally declining hormones but is brought about through hormonal changes from surgery (i.e., organ removal) or radiation therapy.  Menopausal symptoms, whether natural or artificially induced, are summarized in *Table 39.*

*Table 39.*  Clinical Manifestations of Menopause

| | |
|---|---|
| **Cardiovascular** | Hot flashes, chills, night sweats, palpitations, heat in the chest, palms, and soles, headache, forgetfulness, insomnia, tachycardia |
| **Hormonal** | Mood swings, depression, irritability, vaginal dryness, fatigue, osteoporosis, abnormal uterine bleeding, vaginitis |
| **Gastrointestinal** | Constipation, loose stools, weight gain, loss of appetite, thirst |
| **Musculoskeletal** | Bone, muscle, and joint pain, soreness of the lumbar region, arthralgia, myalgia, hip pain |
| **Neurological** | Tinnitus, dizziness, vertigo |
| **Lymphatic** | Edema of the lower limbs |
| **Urinary** | Urinary incontinence, painful urination, urinary frequency |

*The symptoms listed here have been grouped into the closest categories possible according to the systems. However, as both Western and Oriental healthcare practitioners acknowledge, there can be multiple causes for any problem.  This list is not intended to suggest treatment.*

Western therapy includes psychological and physiological treatment.  When psychological symptoms predominate, counseling and/or mild antidepressants are often prescribed.  For physiological symptoms, especially hot flashes (which can continue for years), estrogen replacement therapy (ERT) is a commonly recommended option. Replacement therapy keeps naturally declining hormonal levels at the premeno-pausal level and as a result, menses continues.

Estrogen therapy has the benefit of reducing hot flashes, but as with most Western medication, it is not without its side effects and/or contraindications, which physicians use to evaluate the suitability of this therapy for specific patients. The responsible healthcare pro-vider should point these out to the prospective candi-date. For comparison purposes, the indications and contraindications of ERT are summarized in *Table 40*.

*Table 40.* Benefits and Risks of Estrogen Replacement Therapy (ERT)

| | |
|---|---|
| **Benefits** | Substantially reduces hot flashes. |
| | Helps to reduce vaginitis, urinary frequency, painful urination, and incontinence. |
| | Helps to prevent osteoporosis when used with Vitamin D, adequate nutrition, and weight-bearing exercise. |
| | Reduces heart attacks by 33 percent. |
| | When combined with progesterone, decreases risk of uterine cancer. |
| **Risks** | Possible increase in blood pressure (although not associated with cerebrovascular accident). |
| | Possible increase in diseases of the liver and gall bladder. |
| | Fluid retention, kidney stones, uterine cancer. |
| | Manipulation of the normal menstrual cycle by hormonal means. |
| **Contraindications** | History of severe liver disease. |
| | Estrogen-dependent neoplasms of the endometrium. |
| | History of embolisms or phlebitis. |

Although dosages may need modifying from time to time, for women who have turned to ERT, there is usually immediate relief from the symptoms of dryness and hot flashes. However, even for women who can take estrogen, there are still risks and the well-trained and responsible healthcare provider will explain and monitor them. In this approach, the multiple manifes-tations of menopause are managed primarily by chemi-cal intervention.

# The Chinese Clinical Perspective

In Chapter One of the Su Wen, the first book of the *Neijing* and perhaps the oldest medical text in any tradition, the "Qi cycle" or the Pattern of Female Growth and Development is discussed. This cycle is presented in diagram form in *Table 41*.

| | |
|---|---|
| Age 7 | The Kidney qi becomes abundant, the hair begins to grow longer, the teeth begin to change. |
| Age 14 | The Ren Mai begins to flow, the heaven cycle begins, the Chong Mai begins to grow in abundance, menstruation begins, pregnancy is possible. |
| Age 21 | The Kidney qi becomes equal (i.e., the yin/yang are balanced), the wisdom teeth begin to grow. |
| Age 28 | The tendons, muscles, bones become hard, the hair grows to the longest, the body and mind are in top condition. |
| Age 35 | The Yangming meridians begin to weaken, with the result that the complexion starts to wither, the hair begins to fall off. |
| Age 42 | The three yang meridians of the hands and legs begin to weaken, the complexion looks even more withered, the hair turns gray. |
| Age 49 | The Ren Mai becomes deficient, the heaven cycle becomes exhausted, the Chong Mai becomes weakened and scanty, the body becomes old and cannot become pregnant. |

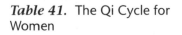

+ = Increases
– = Declines

| 7 | 14 | 21 | 28 | 35 | 42 | 49 |
|---|---|---|---|---|---|---|
| KI qi+ | Ren Mai+ Chong Mai+ Heaven Cycle+ | KI qi equal | Top Condition | Yangming– | Three yang of leg and hands– | Ren Mai– Chong Mai– Heaven Cycle– |

***Table 41.*** The Qi Cycle for Women

According to the Su Wen, we can see that the physiological decline of the essential substances begins after the apogee of a woman's health at about age twenty-eight. By age thirty-five, the Yangming meridians (Stomach and Large Intestine), which contribute to the formation of postnatal qi and blood, begin to decline. The complexion begins to wither (dry/dull/wrinkle) and the hair starts to fall out. These symptoms all indicate blood, qi, yin, and jing deficiency.

By age forty-two, all the yang organs have become weak, the face darkens, and the hair turns gray. These are further indications of insufficiency of the essential substances. By age forty-nine the Directing Vessel (Ren Mai) is empty, the Penetrating Vessel (Chong Mai, Sea of Blood) is depleted, the dew of heaven (menses) dries up, the Earth Passage (uterus) is not open, and weakness and infertility set in.

When the Ren and Chong channels become deficient and the Kidney qi declines, the dew of heaven correspondingly dries up. Kidney qi deficiency means that both the yin and the yang are impaired, and it is evident that this is the basis for the clinical manifestations of menopause. This deficiency of yin and yang expresses itself as hot and cold symptoms. However, it is important that the individual signs and symptoms not be treated independently, but be blended into a whole that differentiates the pattern so that the practitioner will be able to decide on a treatment.

The Chinese literature does not say that women will develop all the signs and symptoms presented here and that are commonly known as the menopausal syndrome. Although all women will experience a decline, particularly in the function of Kidney qi, some women stop having their periods with little or no discomfort. As the Su Wen indicates, at about the same age that menopause in women is diagnosed by Western physicians, menopause occurs according to Chinese medicine as well. This is because of the natural rise and fall of the qi of the body's organs, meridians, and essential substances. Similar signs and symptoms are experienced by many women.

What accounts for the pathological development of such a wide range in the intensity of these symptoms? From a Chinese medical perspective, these disharmonies are a direct reflection of the overall condition of the woman's vital qi. As a result, the more ample the qi and blood, and the healthier the woman's Kidney energy, the less likely it is that she will experience menopausal symptoms. The greater the deficiency, the greater the likelihood that there will be symptoms affecting almost every organ's sphere of influence. The intensity of the experience will be a direct function of her underlying weaknesses. This mechanism is illustrated in *Table 42*.

***Table 42.*** Health of a Woman Undergoing the "Change of Life"

| |
|---|
| The greater the integrity of the essential substances (qi, blood, shen, jing, jin-ye and marrow), the greater the ease of menopause. This leads to normal symptoms such as the loss of the period. Other symptoms are minimal. |
| The weaker the integrity of the essential substances, the greater the difficulty of menopause. This leads to abnormal symptoms (see Table 39). The number and intensity of the symptoms is a direct function of the underlying deficiency. |

Premature menopause in Chinese medicine would also be considered a direct function of the condition of the woman's qi and blood. If qi and blood are weakened from factors such as chemotherapy, which consumes the blood and yin, or surgery, which can cause trauma to organs and blockages in meridian pathways, menopause may be early. Thus, both menopause and menstruation offer women a direct way of knowing more about the condition of their vital energy.

This mechanism asserts that the qualitative experience of menopause is based on the person's predisposing health, or what would be called in Chinese medicine the "host energy." Given this hypothesis, we can be almost sure that if a woman has had a history of menstrual problems, she can expect to have a difficult time with menopause. These symptoms include amenorrhea, dysmenorrhea, cramps, clots, headaches, breast distention and/or tenderness, fibroids, cysts, backaches, abdominal pain, neck tension, fatigue, feeling cold at the time of the period, emotional lability, depression, moodiness, and irritability (symptoms commonly referred to as PMS). There can also be cravings for spicy foods, coffee (or other qi decongesters), sugar, chocolate, alcohol (which temporarily relaxes the Liver), or salt. The earlier this predisposition can be assessed and treated, the greater the likelihood that this dreaded and uncomfortable disorder can be avoided.

On the other hand, women who have been virtually asymptomatic throughout most of their gynecological and obstetric history can almost be assured that menopause will pass easily. And of course, the reason why so many women do have problems with their cycle stems from many factors. These can include dietary problems, stress, overwork, drug use (including coffee, alcohol, recreational and prescription drugs, and birth control pills), to name some of the more common causes. The effects of these etiological factors lead to yin deficiency—Kidney qi xu—and Liver yin and blood deficiency.

The differentiations of menopause can be described in zang-fu terms and tend to cluster around the patterns of disharmony that involve Kidney qi xu, Liver qi stagnation and yin deficiency, and Spleen and Heart blood deficiency. However, for best results, each woman should always be considered as unique.

# The Treatment of Menopause

As Chapters Eleven and Twelve of this book point out, menopause responds well to the Master (Confluent) points of the Eight Curious Vessels. The reasons include the following:

1. The Eight Curious Vessels are rich reservoirs of jing. As such, they are capable of supplementing the organism with jing. As we have seen, certain menopausal symptoms are a reflection of the amount of jing qi that one has.

2. Because of their unique ability to absorb perverse pathogens, the Eight Curious Vessels can treat the symptoms associated with fire and blood stasis, good examples of perversity.

3. As homeostatic vessels, they are capable of regulating physiological fluctuations in the woman.

4. With their ability to nourish the extraordinary organs as well as the hepatobiliary system, the Curious Vessels will obviously have an effect on the uterus and the Dai channel, which in turn will have consequences for the manifestations of menopause.

5. The Curious Vessels regulate the qi and blood of the twelve main meridians. They thus command and supervise various parts of the body and its functions.

6. Because of their intersections with the twelve main meridians the Eight Curious Vessels can be used when the twelve main meridians have failed.

7.  When many deficiencies point in the same direction (in this case Kidney qi xu, Spleen and Heart qi and blood deficiency, Liver blood and yin deficiency and jing deficiency), the Eight Curious Vessels may be used.

8.  They also can be used to treat the root cause of the disease.

Chapter Twelve describes the clinical energetics of the Master and Coupled points of the Eight Curious Vessels.  Refer also to the Eight Confluent point protocol in *Table 28* (found in Chapter Eleven), which outlines needling directions, palpation, and needling sensations.

Within the repertoire of Chinese medicine, there are herbal formulations to address symptoms of Kidney yin and yang xu, as well as the symptoms of menopause.  Because pathological menopause is essentially a reflection of deficiency, menopausal patients should be treated with Chinese herbs to provide them with substantive, biological support.

In an effort to enhance patient compliance with taking herbs, I prescribed many Chinese patent formulas instead of customized formulas. (Remember that many of these patients do not take the time to eat right, let alone prepare decoctions.)  Because these formulas had little effect, I searched for good quality American products that combine Chinese herbs with nutritional supplements.  Three products, all from Metagenics, became my products of choice for menopausal patients and produced excellent results.  I also used a Chinese product known as Recovery of Youth or Green Vitality Treasure.  These products were so effective that many patients did not require any acupuncture, only herbal therapy.  The products, their constituents, and their energetics are discussed below.  Suppliers' addresses are also provided.

## 1. Fem-Estro

### Differentiation
Menopausal complaints from Kidney qi xu, Liver yin deficiency, and Liver yang rising.

### Ingredients
- Vitamin E (d-alpha tocopherol succinate)
- Radix ginseng (Korean)
- Bioflavonoids (undiluted)
- Vitamin B5 (calcium d-pantothenate)
- PABA (para-aminobenzoic acid)
- Vitamin C (corn-free ascorbic acid)
- Raw adrenal concentrate

### Energetics of Ingredients[1]
*Vitamin E* is a yang tonic. It nourishes Liver Blood and tonifies Kidney Yang. It benefits jing, and nourishes the sinews.

*Korean ginseng* tonifies the qi and strengthens the yang. It goes to the Dan Tian and tonifies the prenatal qi.

*Bioflavonoids* regulate the blood, clear heat from the Liver, and stop bleeding.

*Vitamin B5* regulates the qi, relieves Liver qi stagnation, harmonizes the Liver, Spleen, and Stomach, raises the yang, and clears and eliminates damp-heat.

*PABA* tonifies the Liver and Kidneys, nourishes the blood and benefits the jing. It moistens the intestines and promotes bowel movements. It expels wind from the skin, blackens the hair, and retards aging.

*Vitamin C* clears heat, stops bleeding, dissolves toxins, clears heat from the Heart, and calms the shen.

*Raw adrenal concentrate* nourishes the Liver and Kidneys, tonifies Kidney qi and clears deficiency heat.

The effect of this formula is to provide the biological, nutritional basis for female metabolism during menopause. Its unique blend of vitamins, food concen-

---

1. Flaws B: *TCM Description of Fem Estro Rx* (available from Metagenics).

trates, bioflavonoids and herbs is formulated to provide the coenzymes needed in the production and metabolism of hormones. It was designed to provide nutritional support for women with low estrogen levels especially during menopause.

## Dosage
One tablet four times a day.

## Comments
Dosages need to be adjusted. Even in the most complicated cases of menopause, the maximum number of tablets that I have prescribed has been three: one in the morning, one at noon, and one in midafternoon. I have found that if a tablet is taken too late in the afternoon, the patient may develop insomnia, probably from the ginseng and B vitamins. Many patients have been able to control the symptoms of menopause, especially the hot flashes, with just one tablet in the morning. The general rule of thumb I have formulated has been that the greater the deficiency as manifested through the number and intensity of symptoms, the more tablets the patient requires. The earlier the symptoms develop, and the faster they are addressed, the fewer tablets are needed. The patient's need to continue to take the product will be determined by her symptoms. In my experience, this could be for several years. I view taking the herbs as taking food, not as dependence on a drug. In this way the patient can receive solid nutritional supplementation.

## 2. Multigenics

## Ingredients
- Beta-carotene
- Vitamin A (palmitate)
- Vitamin E (d-alpha tocopherol succinate)
- Vitamin D (cholecalciferol)
- Vitamin C (corn-free ascorbic acid)
- Aspartic acid (mineral aspartates)

- Niacinamid
- Trimethylglycine HCl
- Choline (bitartrate)
- Inositol
- Pantothenic acid (calcium pantothenate)
- Bioflavonoids
- PABA (para-amino benzoic acid)
- Vitamin B6 (pyridoxine HCl)
- Vitamin B2 (riboflavin)
- Vitamin B1 (thiamin mononitrate)
- Niacin
- Folic acid
- Biotin
- Vitamin B12 (cyanocobalamin)
- Calcium (citrate)
- Magnesium (glycinate) equivalent in bioavailability to 400 milligrams magnesium (oxide)
- Potassium (aspartate)
- Iron (glycinate)
- Zinc (aspartate)
- Manganese (aspartate)
- Copper (rice amino acid chelate)
- Chromium (nicotinate glycinate)
- Selenium (aspartate)
- Iodine (potassium iodide)
- Molybdenum (aspartate)
- Vanadyl sulfate

In most people's opinion the purpose of a multivitamin is to provide the most complete formula of all the important nutrients in the most absorbable form. Such is the case with this formula.

## Dosage
For adults, one to six tablets daily.

## Comments
The number of tablets to take daily depends on the

degree of nutritional deficiency the patient has. The product is best taken with meals instead of on an empty stomach. A modification of this formula without iron is available from the same company; another is available without iron and copper. Multigenics is particularly effective for menopausal patients with past or current poor nutritional habits.

## 3. Cal-Apatite

### Ingredients
- Microcrystalline Hydroxyapatite
- Elemental Calcium
- Phosphorus
- Trace minerals: Magnesium, Zinc, Potassium, Mangenese, Iron, and others
- Protein as collagen (Glysosaminoglycans and substitute amino acids)

### Dosage
Three to six tablets daily in divided doses.

### Comments
Metagenics claims that tests have shown a significant increase in bone mass with this product. It is extremely well-absorbed. In the case of menopause, it is recommended for the woman who is either worried about future bone loss or who has actually experienced a diminution of bone density.

The patient in *Case 9* (see Chapter Twelve) was prescribed the three products listed above. They definitively contributed to her improvement.

## 4. Ching Chun Bao (Qing Chun Bao): Recovery of Youth Tablets, Antiaging Tablets, Green Vitality Treasure

### Ingredients
Contains at least twenty herbs, many of which are not listed on the label. The main ingredients, however, are ginseng root, asparagus root, and rehmannia root.

## Energetics

Postpones aging, maintains youthful face, and enhances youthful vigor. Strengthens Kidney yang, tonifies qi and blood, promotes blood circulation, benefits the Heart and Kidney, enriches sexual function, counters fatigue. Tonic for aged and debilitated patients. Useful for poor memory, senility, poor resistance to disease, and for strengthening the heart.[2]

## Dosage

Twice a day, three to five tablets each time.

## Comments

My recommendation is to take one dose in the morning and one before going to bed. This is a fabulous product. Take for one month at a time. May be repeated as needed.

I frequently prescribe all of the four products listed above to premenopausal and menopausal patients. They experience excellent results.

## Product Information

### Fem-Estro, Multigenics, and Cal-Apatite

Metagenics
12445 East 39th Avenue, Suite 400
Denver, CO 80239
Tel: (303) 371-6848

### Antiaging Tablets

Mayway Trading Company
622 Broadway, San Francisco, CA 94133
Tel: (415) 788-3946

---

2. Fratkin J: *Chinese Herbal Patent Medicines, A Practical Guide.* Institute for Traditional Medicine and Preventive Health Care, Portland, Ore., 1986; p 190.

# CHAPTER 19

# EPILOGUE

The Heart of the Acupuncturist,
The Heart of the Healer,
The Heart of the Being

The best lesson and the greatest wisdom of this book are in the ancient knowledge that has inspired it. The personal philosophy that follows may help put into perspective the spirit of how to use this manual. As an acupuncturist, striving to become an effective healer, the healer that you already are, the healer that resides within your heart, you may find my approach useful.

I have discussed throughout this work the fact that the delivery of healthcare within the Chinese medical model requires us to carefully observe the human condition. We must categorize and understand every facet of the information from the interview and the examination process. We must perceive the etiology and pathogenesis of signs and symptoms and weave them into a whole that represents the unique constellation of energy of each person. We must blend these pieces of information into a pattern of interaction that aptly describes the individual as energy in motion, a specific expression of the life force.

Although the ability to discern patterns is fundamental to understanding the patient's "dis-ease," we must combine this ability with the appropriate tools and techniques that are the instruments of cure and prevention. The dual ability to diagnose and to treat is crucial to affecting the change that is the fundamental goal of Chinese medicine. But without the ability to be with the patient, to respond to the person's immediate presence with compassion, treatment will only be a deductive, mechanical process. If we cannot grasp the spirit of the patient with our whole being, we will probably fail to reach them with the needle. We will not have grasped the tiger's tail.

The "heavenly," intellectual skills of thinking, reasoning, and learning can be taught. So, too, can the "earthly" ones of manipulating the needle and effortlessly sinking it into the patient's body to encounter the qi. But between these two realms is the place of "man," the place that the body and the spirit inhabits. It is here that we can diagnose and see the patterns of interaction. We can feel the gross and subtle life force of our patients if we bring the fullness of our humanity to the patient-practitioner relationship.

If the heavenly and earthly skills do not merge in us, if the techniques cannot be an expression of the treatment plan, good therapeutic results and personal satisfaction probably will not be achieved. But if these skills melt together through the medium of our humanity, in the place of our hearts, as effortlessly as yin and yang, each will be different and less distinct, as the heavenly and earthly follow and modify each other. We will know not only what to treat, but how to treat. And, we will know how to balance the knowledge of the human condition with the tools for its correction and growth once our mutual human spirit becomes the medium for redressing imbalances.

If we open our hearts to the energy of our patients and the energy of our discipline, our mutual life forces have the opportunity to meet and connect. This union is "the way in," a two-way street, the Tao. It is the way to grasp the essence of the person and for us to capture its spirit, to redirect and root it.

Without the "spiritual" connection of two entities reaching out to each other, which is the natural tendency of our hearts, the essence of what to do, how to do it, and the permission to do it may never be achieved.  This indeed is the tiger's tail.  That magical, powerful, potent animal, seemingly so elusive, is within our grasp—if we adopt the heart of the acupuncturist, the heart of the healer, which is the heart of our being.

TRANSLATIONS OF THE POINT NAMES
SUBJECT INDEX
DISEASE INDEX
POINT INDEX
GLOSSARY
BIBLIOGRAPHY
BIOGRAPHICAL NOTES

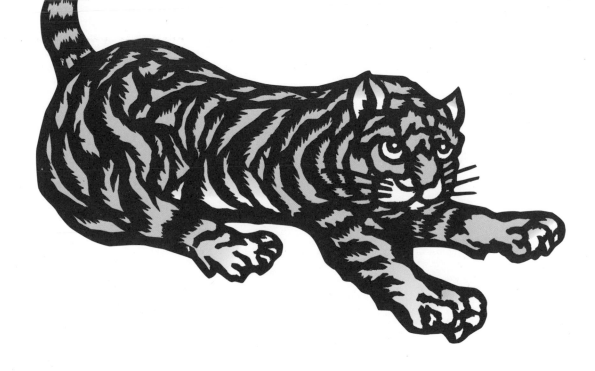

## Translations of the Point Names

*The column on the left (Chinese name and literal translation) gives the Chinese name for each meridian, followed by the exact English word translation underneath it. For example, in the first entry: "Zhong" means "Middle" and "fu" means "place."*

### Lung Meridian

| | CHINESE NAME AND LITERAL TRANSLATION | FIGURATIVE TRANSLATION |
|---|---|---|
| LU 1 | Zhong • fu<br>Middle • place | Central dwelling |
| LU 2 | Yun • men<br>Cloud • door | Gate of the clouds |
| LU 3 | Tian • fu<br>Heaven • place | Celestial dwelling |
| LU 4 | Xia • bai<br>Same as • white | White of the arms |
| LU 5 | Chi • ze<br>A unit of length • marsh | Pool of the arms |
| LU 6 | Kong • zui<br>Opening • adverb | Deep emergence |
| LU 7 | Lie • que<br>Arrangement • depression | Succession of lightning flashes |
| LU 8 | Jing • qu<br>Passing • ditch | Channel emission |
| LU 9 | Tai • yuan<br>Maximum • abyss | Extreme abyss |
| LU 10 | Yu • ji<br>Fish • border | Border of the fish |
| LU 11 | Shao • shang<br>Immaturity • one of the five sounds related to metal | Yang exchange |

### Large Intestine Meridian

| | | |
|---|---|---|
| LI 1 | Shang • yang<br>Maximum • abyss | Exchange of yang |
| LI 2 | Er • jian<br>Second • clearance | Second zone |
| LI 3 | San • jian<br>Third • clearance | Third zone |
| LI 4 | He • gu<br>Junction • valley | Convergence of valleys |
| LI 5 | Yang • xi<br>Opposite of yin • ditch | Torrent of yang |
| LI 6 | Pian • li<br>Divergence • passway | Passage to the side of the mountain |
| LI 7 | Wen • liu<br>Warming • circulation | Balanced flow |
| LI 8 | Xia • lian<br>Inferior • edge | Lower border |
| LI 9 | Shang • lian<br>Superior • edge | Upper border |
| LI 10 | Shou • san • li<br>Upper limbs • numeral • cun in ancient times | Three measures |
| LI 11 | Qu • chi<br>Crooked • pond | Sloped pool |

| | | **Large Intestine Meridian cont.** |
|---|---|---|
| LI 12 | Zhou • liao<br>Elbow • seam | Elbow bone |
| LI 13 | Shou • wu • li<br>Upper limbs • numeral • cun<br>in ancient times | Five measures |
| LI 14 | Bi • nao<br>Upper limbs • arm muscle<br>              prominence | Arm |
| LI 15 | Jian • yu<br>Shoulder • corner | Shoulder bone |
| LI 16 | Ju • gu<br>Big • bone | Giant bone |
| LI 17 | Tian • ding<br>Heaven • name of an ancient utensil | Celestial vase |
| LI 18 | Fu • tu<br>Nearby • prominence | Supporting prominence |
| LI 19 | Kou • he • liao<br>Mouth • grain • seam | Bone of the cereals |
| LI 20 | Ying • xiang<br>Welcome • fragrance | Reception of odors |

| | | **Stomach Meridian** |
|---|---|---|
| ST 1 | Cheng • qi<br>Receiving • tears | Receives the tears |
| ST 2 | Si • bai<br>Four directions • brightness | Four emptiness |
| ST 3 | Ju • liao<br>Great • seam | Giant bone |
| ST 4 | Di • cang<br>Earth • granary | Earth granary |
| ST 5 | Da • ying<br>Opposite of small • welcome | Great reception |
| ST 6 | Jia • che<br>Cheek • vehicle | Maxilla |
| ST 7 | Xia • guan<br>Lower • pass | Lower barrier |
| ST 8 | Tou • wei<br>Head • corner | Cranial suture |
| ST 9 | Ren • ying<br>Mankind • welcome | Meeting with man |
| ST 10 | Shui • tu<br>Water-grain • passing | Rushing water |
| ST 11 | Qi • she<br>Air • residence | Lodge of the energy |
| ST 12 | Que • pen<br>Depression • name of a utensil | Supraclavicular fossa |
| ST 13 | Qi • hu<br>Air • door | Door of the energy |
| ST 14 | Ku • fang<br>Storehouse • side room | House of treasure |
| ST 15 | Wu • yi<br>Room • screening | House screen |
| ST 16 | Ying • chuang<br>Chest • window | Window of the chest |
| ST 17 | Ru • zhong<br>Nipple • middle | Center of the breast |

## Stomach Meridian cont.

| ST 18 | Ru • gen<br>Nipple • root | Base of the breast |
|---|---|---|
| ST 19 | Bu • rong<br>Do not • containing | Does not contain |
| ST 20 | Cheng • man<br>Standing • fullness | Contains the fullness |
| ST 21 | Liang • men<br>Grain • door | Gate to the upper part |
| ST 22 | Guan • men<br>Pass • door | Barrier of the gate |
| ST 23 | Tai • yi<br>Maximum • one of the ten Heavenly Stems | Venus |
| ST 24 | Hua • rou • men<br>Fine • muscle • door | Gate to the slippery flesh |
| ST 25 | Tian • shu<br>Heaven • pivot | Celestial hinge |
| ST 26 | Wai • ling<br>Opposite of interior • hill | External mound |
| ST 27 | Da • ju<br>Opposite of small • great | Giant |
| ST 28 | Shui • dao<br>Water • passage | Canalization of water |
| ST 29 | Gui • lai<br>Return • arrival | Cyclic return |
| ST 30 | Qi • chong<br>Meridian • pass | Assault of energy |
| ST 31 | Bi • guan<br>Thigh • joint | Coxofemoral barrier |
| ST 32 | Fu • tu<br>Sleeping posture • rabbit | Concealed rabbit |
| ST 33 | Yin • shi<br>Opposite of yang • market | Yin trading center |
| ST 34 | Liang • qiu<br>Ridge of a hill • mound | Connecting hill |
| ST 35 | Du • bi<br>Small cow • nose | Calf's nostril |
| ST 36 | Zu • san • li<br>Lower limbs • numeral • used | Three measures on the leg |
| ST 37 | Shang • ju • xu<br>Upper • great • void | Edge of the upper part |
| ST 38 | Tiao • kou<br>Long strip • clearance | End of the tendon |
| ST 39 | Xia • ju • xu<br>Lower • great • void | Edge of the lower part |
| ST 40 | Feng • long<br>Plentiful • abundance | The thunder |
| ST 41 | Jie • xi<br>Separation • stream | Released stream |
| ST 42 | Chong • yang<br>Pass • opposite of yin | Assault of yang |
| ST 43 | Xian • gu<br>Depression • valley | Deep valley |
| ST 44 | Nei • ting<br>Interior • court | Inner courtyard |
| ST 45 | Li • dui<br>Stomach • door | Controlled exchange |

## Spleen Meridian

| SP 1 | Yin • bai<br>Hidden • white | Hidden emptiness |
|------|------|------|
| SP 2 | Da • du<br>Big • infusion | Great center |
| SP 3 | Tai • bai<br>Maximum • white | Venus |
| SP 4 | Gong • sun<br>Connection • reticular collateral | Ancestor and descendant |
| SP 5 | Shang • qiu<br>One of the five sounds<br>related to metal • mound | Hill of exchange |
| SP 6 | Sanyin • jiao<br>Three yin meridians • crossing | Junction of the three yin |
| SP 7 | Lou • gu<br>Point opening • valley | Sleeping valley |
| SP 8 | Di • ji<br>Earth • importance | Earth's vitality |
| SP 9 | Yin • ling • quan<br>Opposite of yang • hill • spring | Source of the yin hill |
| SP 10 | Xue • hai<br>Blood • sea | Sea of blood |
| SP 11 | Ji • men<br>Dustpan • door | Woven basket's outlet |
| SP 12 | Chong • men<br>Pass • door | Gate of the assault |
| SP 13 | Fu • she<br>Zang-fu • dwelling | Warehouse |
| SP 14 | Fu • jie<br>Abdomen • stagnation | Knot of the abdomen |
| SP 15 | Da • heng<br>Large • opposite of vertical | Great transversal |
| SP 16 | Fu • ai<br>Abdomen • pain | Abdominal suffering |
| SP 17 | Shi • dou<br>Food • hole | Reserve of nourishment |
| SP 18 | Tian • xi<br>Heaven • stream | Celestial stream |
| SP 19 | Xiong • xiang<br>Chest • window | Region of the chest |
| SP 20 | Zhou • rong<br>General • nourishment | Pasture of the vital energy |
| SP 21 | Da • bao<br>Major • containing | Great envelope |

## Heart Meridian

| HT 1 | Ji • quan<br>Very high • spring | Extreme source |
|------|------|------|
| HT 2 | Qing • ling<br>Origination • diety | Spirit of azure |
| HT 3 | Shao • hai<br>Immaturity • sea | Young sea |
| HT 4 | Ling • dao<br>Mind • pathway | Spiritual path |
| HT 5 | Tong • li<br>Relation • interior | Path of communication |

## Heart Meridian cont.

| HT 6 | Yin • xi<br>Opposite of yang • cleft | Deep issuance of yin |
|------|--------------------------------------|----------------------|
| HT 7 | Shen • men<br>Mind • door | Gate of spirit |
| HT 8 | Shao • fu<br>Youthful • gathering place | Young dwelling |
| HT 9 | Shao • chong<br>Youthful • impulse | Young assault |

# Small Intestine Meridian

| SI 1 | Shao • ze<br>Small • marsh | Young marsh |
|------|----------------------------|-------------|
| SI 2 | Qian • gu<br>Opposite of back • valley | Anterior valley |
| SI 3 | Hou • xi<br>Opposite of front • ditch | Superior torrent |
| SI 4 | Wan • gu<br>Wrist • bone | Wrist bone |
| SI 5 | Yang • gu<br>Opposite of yin • valley | Valley of yang |
| SI 6 | Yang • lao<br>Nourishing • old | Generates the aged |
| SI 7 | Zhi • zheng<br>Divergence • regular meridian | Straight branch |
| SI 8 | Xiao • hai<br>Small • sea | Small sea |
| SI 9 | Jian • zhen<br>Shoulder • first | Reliable shoulder |
| SI 10 | Noa • shu<br>Upper arm • point | Point of the arm |
| SI 11 | Tian • zong<br>The upper part • respect | Origin of heaven |
| SI 12 | Bing • feng<br>Receiving • pathogenic wind | Catches the wind |
| SI 13 | Qu • yuan<br>Crooked • wall | Inclined ruin |
| SI 14 | Jian • wai • shu<br>Shoulder • lateral aspect • point | External point of the shoulder |
| SI 15 | Jian • zhong • shu<br>Shoulder • interior • point | Central point of the shoulder |
| SI 16 | Tian • chuang<br>Upper part • window | Celestial window |
| SI 17 | Tian • rong<br>Upper part • abundance | Glimpse of heaven |
| SI 18 | Quan • liao<br>Cheek • seam | Zygomatic bone |
| SI 19 | Ting • gong<br>Hearing • palace | Palace of the hearing |

# Bladder Meridian

| BL 1 | Jing • ming<br>Eye • brightness | Clarity of the eye |
|------|---------------------------------|--------------------|
| BL 2 | Zan • zhu<br>Gathered • bamboo | Bore of bamboo |

| BL 3 | Mei • chong<br>Eyebrow • upward | Eyebrow assault |
|------|------|------|
| BL 4 | Qu • chai<br>Crooked • unevenness | Diffferent direction |
| BL 5 | Wu • chu<br>Fifth • place | Five regions |
| BL 6 | Cheng • guang<br>Receiving • brightness | Receives the light |
| BL 7 | Tong • tian<br>Reaching • heaven | Communication with heaven |
| BL 8 | Luo • que<br>Relation • return | Destination of vessels |
| BL 9 | Yu • zhen<br>Jade • pillow | Jade pillow |
| BL 10 | Tian • zhu<br>Heaven • pillar | Pillar of heaven |
| BL 11 | Da • zhu<br>Opposite of small • reed | Great shuttle |
| BL 12 | Feng • men<br>Pathogenic wind • door | Gate of the wind |
| BL 13 | Fei • shu<br>Lung • infusion | Point of the Lung |
| BL 14 | Jueyin • shu<br>End of two yin meridians • infusion | Point of the Jueyin |
| BL 15 | Xin • shu<br>Heart • infusion | Point of the Heart |
| BL 16 | Du • shu<br>Du meridian • infusion | Point of the Du Mai |
| BL 17 | Ge • shu<br>Diaphragm • infusion | Point of Diaphragm |
| BL 18 | Gan • shu<br>Liver • infusion | Point of Liver |
| BL 19 | Dan • shu<br>Gall bladder • infusion | Point of Gall Bladder |
| BL 20 | Pi • shu<br>Spleen • infusion | Point of Spleen |
| BL 21 | Wei • shu<br>Stomach • infusion | Point of Stomach |
| BL 22 | Sanjiao • shu<br>Sanjiao • infusion | Point of Triple Heater |
| BL 23 | Shen • shu<br>Kidney • infusion | Point of Kidney |
| BL 24 | Qihai • shu<br>Sea of primary Qi • infusion | Point of primary Qi |
| BL 25 | Dachang • shu<br>Large intestine • infusion | Point of Large Intestine |
| BL 26 | Guan • yuan • shu<br>Storage • primary Qi • infusion | Point of Qi storage |
| BL 27 | Xiaochang • shu<br>Small intestine • infusion | Point of Small Intestine |
| BL 28 | Pangguang • shu<br>Bladder • infusion | Point of Bladder |
| BL 29 | Zhong • lu • shu<br>Middle • spinal muscle • infusion | Point of the Vertebral Column |
| BL 30 | Bai • huan • shu<br>White • ring • point | Point of the Sphincter |

**Bladder Meridian cont.**

| | | |
|---|---|---|
| BL 31 | Shang • liao<br>Upper • seam | Superior bone |
| BL 32 | Ci • liao<br>Second • seam | Second bone |
| BL 33 | Zhong • liao<br>Middle • seam | Median bone |
| BL 34 | Xia • liao<br>Lower • seam | Inferior bone |
| BL 35 | Hui • yang<br>Crossing • opposite of yin | Meeting of yang |
| BL 36 | Cheng • fu<br>Receiving • support | Maintenance and support |
| BL 37 | Yin • men<br>Thickness • door | Important gate |
| BL 38 | Fu • xi<br>Downstream • hole | Emergence to the surface |
| BL 39 | Wei • yang<br>Crooked • opposite of yin | Yang of the popliteal hollow |
| BL 40 | Wei • zhong<br>Crooked • middle | Popliteal hollow |
| BL 41 | Fu • fen<br>Appending • separation | Supplementary distribution |
| BL 42 | Po • hu<br>Soul • door | Door for entrance of the Po |
| BL 43 | Gao • huang<br>Fat • membrane | Cardio-diaphragmatic region |
| BL 44 | Shen • tang<br>Mind • hall | Hall of all the psychic activities |
| BL 45 | Yi • xi<br>Sighing • sound | Cry of pain |
| BL 46 | Ge • guan<br>Diaphragm • pass | Barrier of the Diaphragm |
| BL 47 | Hun • men<br>Soul • door | Gate for the Hun |
| BL 48 | Yang • gang<br>Opposite of yin • importance | Yang axis |
| BL 49 | Yi • she<br>Emotion • residence | Lodge of the thought |
| BL 50 | Wei • cang<br>Stomach • storehouse | Granary of the Stomach |
| BL 51 | Huang • men<br>Membrane • door | Gate to the cardio-diaphragmatic region |
| BL 52 | Zhi • shi<br>Mind • dwelling | Lodge of the will |
| BL 53 | Bao • huang<br>Bag • membrane | Energetic envelope of the cardio-diaphragmatic region |
| BL 54 | Zhi • bian<br>Order • edge | Beside the border |
| BL 55 | He • yang<br>Confluence • opposite of yin | Reunion of yang |
| BL 56 | Cheng • jin<br>Support • muscle | At the base of the muscle |
| BL 57 | Cheng • shan<br>Support • mountain | At the base of the mountain |
| BL 58 | Fei • yang<br>Flying • opposite of yin | Lightness |

| | **Bladder Meridian cont.** | |
|---|---|---|
| BL 59 | Fu • yang<br>Tarsal • opposite of yin | Supplement of yang |
| BL 60 | Kunlun<br>Name of the mountain | Kunlun mountains |
| BL 61 | Pu • can<br>Servant • paying respects | Serve and consult |
| BL 62 | Shen • mai<br>Extending • meridian | Prolongation of the vessel |
| BL 63 | Jin • men<br>Name of yang • door | Gate of gold |
| BL 64 | Jinggu<br>Ancient name of the tuberosity of<br>the 5th metatarsal | Central bone |
| BL 65 | Shugu<br>Ancient name of the head of<br>the 5th metatarsal | Restrained bone |
| BL 66 | Zu • tong • gu<br>Foot • passing • valley | Communicating valley |
| BL 67 | Zhi • yin<br>Reaching • opposite of yang | Extreme yin |

| | **Kidney Meridian** | |
|---|---|---|
| KI 1 | Yong • quan<br>Gushing • spring | Gushing source |
| KI 2 | Ran • gu<br>Range • valley | Scaphoid tarsus |
| KI 3 | Tai • xi<br>Great • creek | Extreme torrent |
| KI 4 | Da • zhong<br>Opposite of small • heel | Great clock |
| KI 5 | Shui • quan<br>Water • spring | Source of water |
| KI 6 | Zhao • hai<br>Shining • sea | Luminous sea |
| KI 7 | Fu • liu<br>Deep • flowing | Repeated overflow |
| KI 8 | Jiao • xin<br>Crossing • belief | Reunion of the menses |
| KI 9 | Zhu • bin<br>Strong • knee and leg | Constructed riverbank |
| KI 10 | Yin • gu<br>Opposite of yang • valley | Valley of yin |
| KI 11 | Henggu<br>Ancient name of the pubis | Pubic bone |
| KI 12 | Da • he<br>Opposite of small • illustrious | Great agitation |
| KI 13 | Qi • xue<br>Vital energy • room | Point of the energy |
| KI 14 | Si • man<br>Fourth • fullness | Four fullnesses |
| KI 15 | Zhong • zhu<br>Middle • pouring | Central current |
| KI 16 | Huang • shu<br>Membrane • infusion | Point of the cardio-diaphragmatic region |

**Kidney Meridian cont.**

| KI 17 | Shang • qu<br>One of five sounds related to<br>metal • bend | Change of curve |
|---|---|---|
| KI 18 | Shi • guan<br>Stone • importance | Barrier of stone |
| KI 19 | Yin • du<br>Opposite of yang • gathering | Center of the yin |
| KI 20 | Fu • tong • gu<br>Abdomen • passing • water-grain | Communicating valley |
| KI 21 | You • men<br>Deep • door | Pylorus |
| KI 22 | Bu • lang<br>Step • corridor | Corridor |
| KI 23 | Shen • feng<br>Heart • pertaining | Barrier of all the psychic activities |
| KI 24 | Ling • xu<br>Heart • mound | Reunion of the spirituality |
| KI 25 | Shen • cang<br>Heart • housing | Storage of all the psychic activities |
| KI 26 | Yu • zhong<br>Luxuriance • middle | Center of radiation |
| KI 27 | Shu • fu<br>Infusion • fu organ | Center of the points |

## Pericardium Meridian

| PC 1 | Tian • chi<br>Heaven • pool | Celestial pivot |
|---|---|---|
| PC 2 | Tian • quan<br>Heaven • spring | Celestial source |
| PC 3 | Qu • ze<br>Crooked • marsh | Sloped marsh |
| PC 4 | Xi • men<br>Hole • door | Issue from the depth |
| PC 5 | Jian • shi<br>Space • official | Intermediary mediator |
| PC 6 | Nei • guan<br>Interior • pass | Internal barrier |
| PC 7 | Da • ling<br>Big • mound | Great mound |
| PC 8 | Lao • gong<br>Labor • center | Palace of labor |
| PC 9 | Zhong • chong<br>Middle • important place | Central assault |

## Sanjiao (Triple Warmer) Meridian

| TE 1 | Guan • chong<br>Same as bend • important place | Barrier's assault |
|---|---|---|
| TE 2 | Ye • men<br>Water • door | Door for the fluids |
| TE 3 | Zhong • du<br>Middle • water margin | Central island |
| TE 4 | Yang • chi<br>Opposite of yin • pool | Pool of yang |

| TE 5 | Wai • guan<br>External • pass | External barrier |
|------|------------------------------|------------------|
| TE 6 | Zhi • gou<br>Limbs • ditch | Deviated ditch |
| TE 7 | Hui • zong<br>Meeting • gathering | Reunion of the origin |
| TE 8 | Sanyang • luo<br>Three yang meridians of<br>hand • connection | Luo of the three yang |
| TE 9 | Si • du<br>Four • river | Water course |
| TE 10 | Tian • jing<br>Heaven • well | Celestial well |
| TE 11 | Qing • len • zuan<br>Cool • cold • deep water | Cool and clear abyss |
| TE 12 | Xiao • luo<br>Eliminating • soreness, pain, weakness | Vanished river |
| TE 13 | Nao • hui<br>Muscle prominence of the<br>arm • crossing place | Reunion of the arm |
| TE 14 | Jian • liao<br>Shoulder • seam | Shoulder bone |
| TE 15 | Tian • liao<br>Heaven • seam | Heaven's bone |
| TE 16 | Tian • you<br>Heaven • window | Small window of heaven |
| TE 17 | Yi • feng<br>Shielding • pathogenic wind | Wind shield |
| TE 18 | Qi • mai<br>Convulsion • collateral | Enraged vessel |
| TE 19 | Lu • xi<br>Skull • relieving the mind | Cranial transmission |
| TE 20 | Jiao • sun<br>Corner • reticular collateral | Small court |
| TE 21 | Er • men<br>Ear • door | Gate of the ear |
| TE 22 | Er • he • liao<br>Ear • harmony • seam | Osseous reunion |
| TE 23 | Sizhu • kong<br>Thready bamboo • space | Silk bamboo hole |

**Gall Bladder Meridian**

| GB 1 | Tongzi • liao<br>Pupil • seam | Originates from the pupil's bone |
|------|-------------------------------|----------------------------------|
| GB 2 | Ting • hui<br>Hearing • gathering | Reunion of the hearing |
| GB 3 | Shang • guan<br>Upper • border | Upper barrier |
| GB 4 | Han • yan<br>Mandible • obedience | Sluggish chin |
| GB 5 | Xuan • lu<br>Suspended • skull | Suspended skull |
| GB 6 | Xuan • li<br>Suspended • long hair | Suspended minimum |
| GB 7 | Qu • bin<br>Crooked • hair at the temple | Temporal curve |

**Gall Bladder Meridian cont.**

| GB | Chinese / Translation | Meaning |
|---|---|---|
| GB 8 | Shuai • gu<br>Command • valley | Direction of the valley |
| GB 9 | Tian • chong<br>Heaven • important place | Heaven's assault |
| GB 10 | Fu • bai<br>Superficial • white | Floating emptiness |
| GB 11 | Tou • qiao • yin<br>Head • opening • opposite of yang | Yin cavity |
| GB 12 | Wangu<br>Mastoid process of the temporal bone | Mastoid process |
| GB 13 | Ben • shen<br>Essential • mind | Root of all the psychic activities |
| GB 14 | Yang • bai<br>Opposite of yin • brightness | Emptiness of yang |
| GB 15 | Tou • lin • qi<br>Head • regulation • tears | On the verge of tears |
| GB 16 | Mu • chuang<br>Eye • window | Window of the eye |
| GB 17 | Zhengying<br>Fright and fear | Vital energy from the center |
| GB 18 | Cheng • ling<br>Support • mind | Receives the spirituality |
| GB 19 | Nao • kong<br>Brain • cavity | Empty brain |
| GB 20 | Feng • chi<br>Pathogenic wind • pool | Pool of the wind |
| GB 21 | Jian • jing<br>Shoulder • well | Well of the shoulder |
| GB 22 | Yuan • ye<br>Gulf • armpit | Liquids from the depth |
| GB 23 | Zhe • jin<br>Ear of cart (wheel protection plate of the cart) • muscle | Stable muscle |
| GB 24 | Ri • yue<br>Sun • moon | Sun and moon |
| GB 25 | Jing • men<br>Same as "yuan" • door | Gate of the center |
| GB 26 | Dai • mai<br>Waist belt • meridian | Dai mai |
| GB 27 | Wu • shu<br>Five • pivot | Five hinges |
| GB 28 | Wei • dao<br>Maintain • passage | Path of protection |
| GB 29 | Ju • liao<br>Reside • hipbone | Inhabited bone |
| GB 30 | Huan • tiao<br>Circumflexus • leap | Jump of the circle |
| GB 31 | Feng • shi<br>Pathogenic wind • market | Wind trading center |
| GB 32 | Zhong • du<br>Middle • small ditch | Central course of water |
| GB 33 | Xi • yang • guan<br>Knee • opposite of yin • joint | Yang barrier |
| GB 34 | Yang • ling • quan<br>Opposite of yin • mound • spring | Source of the yang hill |
| GB 35 | Yang • jiao<br>Opposite of yin • crossing | External hill |

| | Gall Bladder Meridian cont. |
|---|---|

| GB 36 | Wau • qiu<br>External • mound | Yang intersection |
|---|---|---|
| GB 37 | Guangming<br>Brightness | Bright light |
| GB 38 | Yang • fu<br>Opposite of yin • auxilliary | Yang assistant |
| GB 39 | Xuan • zhong<br>Hanging • bell | Suspended clock |
| GB 40 | Qiu • xu<br>Mound • big mound | Hill trading center |
| GB 41 | Zu • lin • qi<br>Foot • regulation • tears | On the verge of tears |
| GB 42 | Di • wu • hui<br>Ground • five • confluence | Five terrestial reunions |
| GB 43 | Xia • xi<br>Same as "jia" • ditch | Beside the torrent |
| GB 44 | Zu • qiao • yin<br>Foot • opening • opposite of yang | Yin cavity |

## Liver Meridian

| LR 1 | Da • dun<br>Big • thickness | Great calmness |
|---|---|---|
| LR 2 | Xing • jian<br>Walking • middle | Intermediary of movement |
| LR 3 | Tai • chong<br>Same as "da" • important place | Extreme assault |
| LR 4 | Zhong • feng<br>Middle • hidden | Central barrier |
| LR 5 | Li • gou<br>Shell • ditch | Drain of shells |
| LR 6 | Zhong • du<br>Middle • confluence | Central current |
| LR 7 | Xi • guan<br>Knee • joint | Knee barrier |
| LR 8 | Qu • quan<br>Crooked • spring | Curved source |
| LR 9 | Yin • bao<br>Opposite of yang • uterus | Envelope of the yin |
| LR 10 | Zu • wu • li<br>Lower limbs • five • interior | Five measures |
| LR 11 | Yin • lian<br>Opposite of yang • edge | Border of the yin |
| LR 12 | Ji • mai<br>Urgent • artery | Rapid vessel |
| LR 13 | Zhang • men<br>Screen • door | Gate of the section |
| LR 14 | Qi • men<br>Period • door | Gate of the periodic departure |

## Governing Vessel

| GV 1 | Chang • qiang<br>Long • strong | Long strength |
|---|---|---|
| GV 2 | Yao • shu<br>Low back • infusion | Point of the loins |

**Governing Vessel cont.**

| GV 3 | Yao • yang • guan<br>Low back • opposite of yin • joint | Yang barrier |
|------|------|------|
| GV 4 | Ming • men<br>Life • door | Gate of the vitality |
| GV 5 | Xuan • shu<br>Suspended • pivot | Suspended hinge |
| GV 6 | Ji • zhong<br>Spine • middle | Middle of the vertebrae |
| GV 7 | Zhong • shu<br>Middle • pivot | Central hinge |
| GV 8 | Jin • suo<br>Muscle • spasm | Contracted muscles |
| GV 9 | Zhi • yang<br>Reaching • opposite of yin | Extreme yang |
| GV 10 | Ling • tai<br>Spirit • platform | Platform of the spirituality |
| GV 11 | Shen • dao<br>Mind • pathway | Path of all the psychic activities |
| GV 12 | Shen • zhu<br>Body • pillar | Pillar of the body |
| GV 13 | Tao • dao<br>Moulding • way | Ceramic path |
| GV 14 | Da • zhui<br>Big • vertebra | Great vertebrae |
| GV 15 | Ya • men<br>Muteness • door | Gate of muteness |
| GV 16 | Feng • fu<br>Pathogenic wind • place | Dwelling of the wind |
| GV 17 | Noa • hu<br>Brain • door | Entrance door to the brain |
| GV 18 | Qiang • jian<br>Stiffness • middle | Intermediary strength |
| GV 19 | Hou • ding<br>Back • vertex | Posterior vertex |
| GV 20 | Bai • hui<br>Numeral • meeting | A hundred reunions |
| GV 21 | Qian • ding<br>Front • vertex | Anterior vertex |
| GV 22 | Xin • hui<br>Fontanel • closing | Fontanel reunion |
| GV 23 | Shang • xin<br>Upper • star | Upper star |
| GV 24 | Shen • ting<br>Mind • vestibule | Courtyard of all the psychic activities |
| GV 25 | Su • liao<br>Nasal cartilage • seam | Bone of origin |
| GV 26 | Shui • gou<br>Water • groove | Drain |
| GV 27 | Dui • duan<br>Mouth • tip | Extremity of exchange |
| GV 28 | Yin • jiao<br>Gum • junction | Junction with the gum |

## Conception Vessel

| CV 1 | Hui • yin<br>Crossing • genital orifice | Reunion of yin |
|---|---|---|
| CV 2 | Qu • gu<br>Crooked • bone | Pubic bone |
| CV 3 | Zhong • ji<br>Middle • right | Central extremity |
| CV 4 | Guan • yuan<br>Storage • primary qi | Barrier of the origin |
| CV 5 | Shi • men<br>Stone • door | Gate of stone |
| CV 6 | Qi • hai<br>Primary qi • sea | Sea of energy |
| CV 7 | Yin • jiao<br>Opposite of yang • crossing | Intersection of yin |
| CV 8 | Shen • que<br>Spirit • palace door | Umbilicus |
| CV 9 | Shui • fen<br>Water-grain • separation | Division of water |
| CV 10 | Xia • wan<br>Inferior • stomach | Inferior part of the stomach |
| CV 11 | Jian • li<br>Establishing • inferior | Internal construction |
| CV 12 | Zhong • wan<br>Middle • stomach | Central stomach |
| CV 13 | Shang • wan<br>Superior • stomach | Superior part of the stomach |
| CV 14 | Ju • que<br>Great • palace door | Huge tower |
| CV 15 | Jiu • wei<br>Wild pigeon • tail | Turtledove's tail |
| CV 16 | Zhong • ting<br>Middle • court | Central courtyard |
| CV 17 | Tanzhong<br>Pericardium | Sternum |
| CV 18 | Yu • tang<br>Jade • palace | Jade hall |
| CV 19 | Zi • gong<br>Purple • palace | Purple palace |
| CV 20 | Hua • gai<br>Magnificent • umbrella | Flowery covering |
| CV 21 | Xuan • ji<br>Rotation • axis | Precious jade stone |
| CV 22 | Tian • tu<br>Heaven • chimney | Celestial prominence |
| CV 23 | Lian • quan<br>Clear • water spring | Source from the border |
| CV 24 | Cheng • jiang<br>Receiving • water fluid | Receives the liquid |

## Subject Index

## Disease Index

## Point Index

## Large Intestine

## Liver

## Lung

## Pericardium

## Small Intestine

## Extra Points

# Glossary

| | |
|---|---|
| ah shi | Literally means "Oh, yes." These are points that are tender or sensitive when palpated. They do not have definite locations or names |
| Bao gong | The palace or envelope of the child, that is, the uterus |
| Bao luo | An internal vessel that connects the Kidney to the uterus |
| Bao mai | An internal vessel that connects the Pericardium to the uterus |
| Baxie | A set of points located on the dorsum of the hands between each finger at the junction of the margins of the webs |
| Chong Mai | One of the Eight Curious Vessels, the Sea of Blood |
| ci | Thorns on the tongue |
| da qi | The sensation of the arrival of qi, usually to the needle |
| Dai Mai | One of the Eight Curious Vessels, the Belt Vessel |
| Dan Tian | The area in the lower abdomen below the umbilicus that pertains to the Kidney, the root of qi |
| Du Mai | One of the Eight Curious Vessels, the Governing Vessel |
| Erjian | The ear apex point |
| gwa sha | A scraping technique with similar results to bloodletting for the removal of stagnation |
| Huatoujiaji | A group of points on both sides of the spinal column at the lateral borders of the spinous processes of the first thoracic to the fifth lumbar vertebrae |
| jiao | Heater, warmer, burning space |
| jing | Rarefied essence, one of the essential substances |
| Jinjin | One of the veins on the underside of the tongue, located on the frenulum |
| Jueyin | One of the Six Divisions, "the lesser yin" |
| jin-ye | The pure fluids retained by the body for its own use |
| Liu Wei Di Huang Wan | Six Flavor Tea, classical formula for nourishing Kidney and Liver yin and tonifying Kidney and Spleen qi. |

| | |
|---|---|
| luo | Vessel or channel |
| Mai | Meridian, blood vessel |
| Mu | One of the twelve points on the front of the body that pertain to each of the twelve zang-fu organs |
| *Neijing* | The oldest body of Chinese medical literature. Also referred to as *The Yellow Emperor's Classic, The Canon of Acupuncture, The Compendium of Acupuncture and Moxibustion* |
| Possom On | External Chinese medicated ointment that warms the muscles. Good for aches and pains due to injury, stagnant blood or wind-cold |
| qi | Vital energy, the life force |
| Ren Mai | One of the Eight Curious Vessels, the Conception Channel |
| San Jiao | The Triple Warmer, the Triple Heater |
| Shaoyang | The level of the Six Divisions that represents the hinge between the interior and the exterior pertaining to the Gall Bladder and the Triple Warmer |
| Shaoyin | One of the deepest levels of the Six Divisions pertaining to the Heart and Kidney |
| shen | spirit |
| shi | dampness |
| shi tan | dilute phlegm or phlegm-damp |
| Shixuan | A group of points on the tips of the ten fingers |
| Shu | A type of point located on the back medial Bladder line that is associated with the qi of each of the twelve zang-fu organs, as well as other structures |
| Sifeng | On the palmar surface of the hand at the midpoint of the transverse crease of the interphalangeal joints of the index, middle, ring and little fingers |
| Taiyang | The first level of the Six Divisions pertaining to the Bladder and the Small Intestine |
| Taiyin | The fourth level of the Six Divisions pertaining to Lung and Spleen |
| Tieh Ta Yao Gin | External Chinese liniment well known for resolving bruises |
| tan | phlegm |
| Wan Hua | External Chinese liniment to move blood stagnation |

| | |
|---|---|
| wei qi | Protective, defensive qi |
| Xi (cleft) | Point of accumulation or blockage |
| xie qi | Pathogenic energy |
| xin bao | Pericardium (envelope that protects the Heart) |
| xu | Deficiency |
| xue | Originally meaning a cave or a hole, which later became a reference for an acupuncture point; blood |
| Yangqiao Mai | One of the Eight Curious Vessels, the yang heel vessel |
| Yangwei Mai | One of the Eight Curious Vessels, the yang connecting vessel |
| Yangming | One of the Six Division levels, "resplendent sunlight" |
| Yinwei Mai | One of the Eight Curious Vessels, the yin linking channel |
| ying | Nutritive qi |
| Yinqiao Mai | One of the Eight Curious Vessels, the yin heel vessel |
| yuan qi | Source qi, reproductive qi, congenital qi, qi of preheaven, original qi, Kidney qi |
| Yuyue | One of the veins on the underside of the tongue on the frenulum |
| zang-fu | The twelve organs in Chinese medicine |
| Zheng Gu Shui | A powerful external Chinese liniment that penetrates to the bone level and activates qi and blood |

# Bibliography

Almasi MR: The truth about cellulite. *Redbook*. June, 1994.

American Dental Association: Caring for your teeth and gums, 1994.

————: Periodontal Diseases—Don't Wait Till It Hurts. Chicago, 1992.

*Applied Chinese Acupuncture for Clinical Practitioners*. Yuan JQ, Mao GY, and Lin Y (trans). Shandong Science and Technology Press, Shandong, PRC, 1985.

Beijing College of Traditional Chinese Medicine, et al.: *Essentials of Chinese Acupuncture*. Foreign Language Press. Beijing, PRC, 1980.

Berlow R (ed): *The Merck Manual*. Merck and Company, Inc., Rahway, N.J., 15th ed., 1987; 16th ed., 1992.

*Brief Explanation of Acupoints of the 14 Regular Meridians*. Kai Z (trans). Acupoints Research Committee of China, Society of Acupuncture and Moxibustion. Beijing, PRC, 1987.

Christopher J: *School of Natural Healing*. BiWorld Publishers, Inc., Provo, Utah, 1976.

Dale RA: Acupuncture needling: a summary of the principal traditional Chinese methods. *Amer J Acupun*, 1994; 22(2).

Darras JC: *Traite D'Acuponcture Médicale*, Tome I. Barnett M (trans). O.I.C.S. Newsletter, 1982.

Dung HC: Characterization of the three functional phases of acupuncture points. *Chi Med J*, 1984; 97(10).

————: Three principles of acupoints. *Amer J Acupun,* 1984; 12(3).

Flaws B: *Arisal of the Clear, A Simple Guide to Healthy Eating According to Traditional Chinese Medicine*. Blue Poppy Press, Boulder, Colo., 1991.

————: *Free and Easy, Traditional Chinese Acupuncture for American Women*. Blue Poppy Press, Boulder, Colo., 1986.

————: TCM Description of Fem Estro Rx (available from Metagenics).

————: The pill and stagnant blood: the side-effects of oral contraceptives according to traditional Chinese medicine. *J Chi Med*, 1990, 32.

Flaws B (ed): *A Handbook of Traditional Chinese Gynecology*. Blue Poppy Press, Boulder, Colo., 1987.

Flaws B and Wolfe HL: *Prince Wen Hui's Cook, Chinese Dietary Therapy*. Paradigm Press, Brookline, Mass., 1983.

Fratkin J: *Chinese Herbal Patent Medicines, A Practical Guide*. Institute for Traditional Medicine, Portland, Ore., 1986.

Gaeddert A: *Chinese Herbs in the Western Clinic*. Get Well Foundation, Dublin, Calif., 1994.

Gardner-Abbate S: Assessing and treating Pericardium 6 (Neiguan): gate to internal well-being. *Amer J Acupun*, 1995; 23(2).

————: The treatment of periodontal gum disease: a protocol for prevention, maintenance and reversal within the paradigm of traditional Chinese medicine. *Amer J Acupun*, 1995; 23(3).

————: New insight on the etiology and treatment of cellulite according to Chinese medicine: more than skin deep. *Amer J Acupun*, 1995; 23(4).

Hsu H-Y: *Shang Han Lun*. Oriental Healing Arts Institute, Los Angeles, 1981.

Hsu H-Y (ed.): *Natural Healing with Chinese Herbs*. Oriental Healing Arts Institute, Los Angeles, 1982.

Kapit W and Elson L: *The Anatomy Coloring Book*. Barnes and Noble, New York, 1977.

Kaptchuck T: *The Web That Has No Weaver*. Congdon and Weed, New York, 1983.

Kudriavtsev A: Needling methods: translation and commentary on the *Ode to tonification, sedation and clear conscience (Bu xie xu xin ge)* from the "Great Compendium of Acupuncture and Moxibustion" *(Zhen Jiu Da Chang)*. *Amer J Acupun*, 1992; 20(2).

Larée C and Rochat de la Vallee E: The practitioner-patient relationship: wisdom from the Chinese classics. *J Trad Acu*, Winter, 1990-91.

————: *Rooted in Spirit*. Station Hill Press, New York, 1995.

Low R: *The Non-Meridial Points of Acupuncture*. Thorson's Publishing Group, Wellingborough, Northamptonshire, England, 1988.

————: *Acupuncture in Gynecology and Obstetrics*. Thorson's Publishing Group, Wellingborough, Northamptonshire, England, 1990.

Lu H: *Chinese System of Food Cures, Prevention and Remedies*. Sterling Publishing Co., Inc., New York, 1986.

Maciocia G: *The Foundations of Chinese Medicine*. Churchill-Livingston, London, 1989.

————: *Tongue Diagnosis in Chinese Medicine*. Eastland Press, Seattle, 1995.

Matsumoto K: *Extraordinary Vessels*. Paradigm Publications, Brookline, Mass., 1986.

Matsumoto K, Birch S: *Hara Diagnosis, Reflections on the Sea*. Paradigm Publications, Brookline, Mass., 1988.

McGarey W: *Physician's Reference Notebook*. Association for Research and Enlightenment, Virginia Beach, Va., 1968.

Meiquan Z: *The Chinese Plum-Blossom Needle Therapy*. The People's Medical Publishing House, Beijing, PRC, 1984.

Requena Y: *Terrains and Pathology, Vol. 1*. Paradigm Publications, Brookline, Mass., 1986.

————: *Character and Health, The Relationship of Acupuncture and Psychology*. Paradigm Publications, Brookline, Mass., 1989.

Rubik B: Can western science provide a foundation for acupuncture? *Alt Ther,* Sept., 1995; 1(4).

Seem MD: *Acupuncture Imaging, Perceiving the Energy Pathways of the Body*. Healing Arts Press, Rochester, Vt., 1990.

————: TCM versus non-TCM: putting the acupuncture back into Chinese medicine. *J Amer College TCM*, 1989; 7(4).

————: Integrationist acupuncture: plurality in the practice of American acupuncture. *Amer J Acupun*, 1992; 20(3).

Shanghai College of Traditional Chinese Medicine: *Acupuncture, A Comprehensive Text*. Bensky D, O'Connor J (trans/eds). Eastland Press, Chicago, 1981.

*The Treatment of Knotty Diseases with Chinese Acupuncture and Chinese Herbal Medicine*. Gong X and Lian-jun Z (trans). Shandong Science and Technology Press, Shandong, PRC, 1990.

Todd AD: *Double Vision*. University Press of New England, Hanover, N.H., 1994.

Unschuld P: *Medicine in China, A History of Ideas*. University of California Press, Berkeley, 1985.

Wiseman N and Ellis A: *Fundamentals of Chinese Medicine*. Paradigm Publications, Brookline, Mass., 1985.

Wolfe H: *Second Spring, A Guide to Healthy Menopause Through Traditional Chinese Medicine*. Blue Poppy Press, Boulder, Colo., 1990.

World Health Organization: *Standard Acupuncture Nomenclature*, Part 2 (revised). Edited by the Regional Office for the Western Pacific, Manila, 1991.

Youbang C and Liangyue D (eds): *Essentials of Contemporary Chinese Acupuncturists' Clinical Experience*. Foreign Language Press, Beijing, PRC, 1989.

## Abbreviations

*Amer J Acupun*: American Journal of Acupuncture.

*J Amer College TCM*: Journal of the American College of Traditional Chinese Medicine.

*J Trad Acu*: Journal of Traditional Acupuncture.

*J Chi Med*: Journal of Chinese medicine.

*Chi Med J*: Chinese Medical Journal.

# Biographical Notes

Skya Gardner-Abbate, M.A., D.O.M, Dipl.Ac, Dipl.C.H., has served as the Chairman of the Department of Clinical Medicine of Southwest Acupuncture College since 1986. She has also served as a Commissioner on the National Accreditation Commission for Schools and Colleges of Acupuncture and Oriental Medicine for seven years. She holds a master's degree in sociology in addition to her training in traditional Chinese medicine at the Santa Fe College of Natural Medicine (1981–1982), the Institute of Traditional Medicine (1982–1983), and two internships at the International Training Center of the Academy of TCM (1988–1989) in Beijing, PRC.

She is also the author of *Beijing, The New Forbidden City*, a work about her experiences in China at the time of the Tiananmen Square massacre in 1989. Her next book, "The Magic Hand Returns Spring, The Art of Palpatory Diagnosis" is forthcoming in 1997.